EMOTIONAL AND INTERPERSONAL DIMENSIONS
OF HEALTH SERVICES

D1565870

Emotional and Interpersonal Dimensions of Health Services

Enriching the Art of Care with the Science of Care

EDITED BY
LAURETTE DUBÉ
GUYLAINE FERLAND
D.S. MOSKOWITZ

2003

Published for
The McGill Initiative for the Integrative Management of Health
In collaboration with
L'institut universitaire de gériatrie de Montréal
by
McGill-Queen's University Press
Montreal & Kingston · London · Ithaca

Legal deposit fourth quarter 2003
Bibliothèque nationale du Québec

Printed in Canada on acid-free paper that is 100% ancient forest free
(100% post-consumer recycled), processed chlorine free.

McGill-Queen's University Press acknowledges the support of the
Canada Council for the Arts for our publishing program. We also
acknowledge the financial support of the Government of Canada
through the Book Publishing Industry Development Program (BPIDP)
for our publishing activities.

National Library of Canada Cataloguing in Publication

Emotional and interpersonal dimensions of health services: enriching
the art of care with the science of care/edited by Laurette Dubé,
Guylaine Ferland, D.S. Moskowitz.

Papers originally presented at a conference held at the Faculty
of Management, McGill University, May 18-19, 2000.
Includes bibliographical references and index.
ISBN 0-7735-2561-0 (bnd)
ISBN 0-7735-2562-9 (pbk)

1. Medical personnel and patient. 2. Social medicine. 3. Patients–
Psychology. I. Dubé, Laurette II. Ferland, Guylaine, 1957–
III. Moskowitz, Debbie S. IV. Institut universitaire de gériatrie
de Montréal v. McGill Initiative for the Integrative Management
of Health.

R726.5.E42 2003   610.69'6   C2003-902365-6

Typeset in Sabon 10/12
by Caractéra inc., Quebec City

Contents

INTRODUCTION

1 Integrating the Art and Science of Care into the Everyday
Delivery of Health Services: Challenges for Research
and Practice 3
Laurette Dubé, Guylaine Ferland, and D.S. Moskowitz

PART ONE   THE ART OF CARE,
ORGANIZATIONAL CONSTRAINTS, AND
PATIENT AND PROVIDER OUTCOMES

2 Measuring the Quality of the Primary Care Relationship 12
Dana Gelb Safran

3 The Emotional and Interpersonal Dimensions of Health Care
and Their Impact on Organizational and Clinical Outcomes:
Building an Integrative, Action-Oriented Research Agenda 45
Carole A. Estabrooks

4 Measuring and Monitoring Patient Outcomes 55
Diane M. Irvine Doran

PART TWO   THE SCIENCE OF CARE:
FOCUS ON EMOTIONAL PROCESSES

5 Behind Every Great Caregiver: The Emotional Labour in Health
Care 67
Arlie Russell Hochschild

6   Patient Emotions in a Clinical Context: Coping with Anxiety
    and Depression and Other Negative Emotions   73
    Gilbert Pinard

7   Patient Emotions and the "Engineering" of Provider Responses
    for More Effective Care   84
    Laurette Dubé

    PART THREE   THE SCIENCE OF CARE:
    FOCUS ON INTERPERSONAL PROCESSES

8   Interpersonal Process in the Patient-Physician Relationship   98
    Debra L. Roter

9   Patient-Practitioner Communication in Conventional and
    Complementary Medicine Contexts   105
    Heather Boon

10 An Interpersonal Social Support Approach to Understanding the
    Patient-Practitioner Relationship   115
    Krista K. Trobst

    PART FOUR   CHALLENGES IN INTEGRATING
    THE ART AND SCIENCE OF CARE INTO HEALTH
    RESEARCH AND PRACTICE

11 Dynamic Conceptions of Dimensions in the Interpersonal
    Domain   130
    D.S. Moskowitz

12 Methodological Challenges to Capturing Dynamical Aspects of
    Health Care Acquisition   138
    Lawrence R. Levy, Richard W.J. Neufeld, and Weiguang Yao

13 Outcomes in Health Care: Motivation, Measures, and Drivers at
    the Population Level   151
    Terrence Montague

    REFERENCES   163

    CONTRIBUTORS   187

EMOTIONAL AND INTERPERSONAL DIMENSIONS OF HEALTH SERVICES

I

Integrating the Art and Science of Care into the Everyday Delivery of Health Services: Challenges for Research and Practice

LAURETTE DUBÉ, GUYLAINE FERLAND,
D.S. MOSKOWITZ,

Technological and biomedical breakthroughs have given us a remarkable and diverse array of tests, machines, drugs, and procedures for diagnosing and treating diseases ever more effectively, which has translated into improved health status and longevity in modern societies. Such advances have been made possible by the development of a solid theoretical understanding of health, diseases, and medical interventions, supported by a relentless quest for innovation and by extensive, provenly efficacious empirical testing of any new diagnostic or therapeutic intervention. In sharp contrast, modern medicine and professional health practice in general have not taken such strides when it comes to the more human aspects of care, including the interpersonal and emotional processes that are at play between the patient and the provider in each episode of care. Yet Hippocrates' principles bearing on the "art of care" are as relevant today as they have ever been. Particularly as we enter an era of chronic diseases and an aging population, modern practice could benefit from enriching this art through significant developments in the "science of care."

Chronic diseases present unique challenges. In chronic diseases, the provision of professional health services and their effectiveness are intricately linked to an individual's daily life, with quality of care being closely tied to the provider's ability to enable patients to cope more effectively with appropriate daily health behaviours and to seek the support they need from family, community, or official health services. Breakthroughs in managing health in patients with chronic diseases may in the future consist of: (1) a better integration of science-based knowledge of interpersonal and emotional processes into the everyday delivery of care; (2) the empirical testing of the impact of such integration on care outcomes; and (3) the understanding of day-to-day caring from both the patient's and the provider's perspectives. The health and economic payoffs of such efforts have the potential to be high. In Western countries, chronic diseases are estimated to be responsible for 80 per cent of all deaths, and their management consumes 70 per cent of health care expenditures (Hoffman, Rice, and Sung 1996). People aged sixty years and older have, on average, 2.2 chronic conditions (Rothenberg and Koplan 1990).

The focus of this book is on the emotional and interpersonal aspects of health care and their impact on organizational and clinical outcomes. Contributors include scholars interested in basic research on emotions and interpersonal behaviours and others who have pioneered health research on these two core components of the "art of care." The material offered in this book was first presented in a workshop on the emotional and interpersonal aspects of care and their impact on organizational aspects of care. This workshop was funded by the Social Sciences and Humanities Research Council of Canada as part of the Tri-Council Workshop/Networking Program.

THE ART OF CARE, ORGANIZATIONAL CONSTRAINTS, AND PATIENT AND PROVIDER OUTCOMES

Until recently, neither researchers nor practitioners had paid much heed to the degree to which the provision of the "art of care" and its impact on patient outcomes could be conditioned by organizational parameters, such as the administrative structure among stakeholders in the delivery of care or the human resources available for service delivery. Nor has there been much formal assessment of the key mediating role that provider outcomes, such as job satisfaction and conditions in the practice environments, may play in shaping care. The first section of the book presents three chapters by scholars who have each contributed to empirical developments in the area of organizational constraints affecting patient and provider outcomes.

In chapter 2, Dana Gelb Safran demonstrates that emotional and interpersonal processes account for a significant part of patients' perceptions of quality of care and contribute to positive organizational and clinical outcomes in the context of primary care. She and her collaborators identified two "art of care" dimensions – specifically, patients' trust and their perception that they were known as "whole persons" – that were key correlates of three important outcomes of care: adherence to advice concerning health risk factors, satisfaction, and improved health status. The same facets of care also played major roles in determining patients' loyalty to a physician. Results showed that the ability of physicians to provide such "art of care" was dependent on the forms of organizational structure and on the financial arrangements in place in health care systems in which their services were provided.

Carole A. Estabrooks, in chapter 3, focuses on the "art of care" not in terms of how health care providers take care of their patients, but in terms of how health service organizations take care of their staff, namely their nurses. Because the provision of health services involves a purposeful, interpersonal interaction between two human beings, caring for the providers with respect to context, resources, processes, and outcomes is essential. She reports preliminary results from an international study of hospital organization and nurse outcomes conducted in five countries, including Canada (Alberta). The study aims to determine how organizational structures and aspects of the practice environment, such as the team relationship, staffing resources, and nurse control over practice, impact on nurse outcomes (e.g., burnout, job satisfaction). Results indicate that staffing resources in particular have a substantial impact on exhaustion. A nurse in an inadequately staffed environment ends a typical day in the mid-range of emotional exhaustion whereas one whose team is adequately staffed is less emotionally exhausted. The study also finds a high prevalence of psychological and physical abuse in the course of professional practice, with almost half of the nurses reporting some form of abuse during their most recent five shifts.

In chapter 4, Diane Irvine Doran takes the reader one step further with results from a study that examines the impact of nursing-staff job satisfaction on patient outcomes in an acute care setting. From the nurses' perspectives, job satisfaction significantly influences the quality of nursing care as reflected both in the effectiveness of their communication with other health care providers and in the coordination of care. Nurses' satisfaction has direct effects on patient outcomes, such as a patient's functional status, mood disturbances, and ability to self-care. These results suggest that job satisfaction partially mediates the effect of staff and unit structural variables and has a direct effect on the quality of work performance, which in turn affects patients' outcomes.

THE SCIENCE OF CARE:
FOCUS ON EMOTIONAL PROCESSES

Section 2 of the book presents more fundamental research on the emotional dimensions of health care. In chapter 5, Arlie Russell Hochschild, who coined the term "emotional labour" to capture the human dimension of what is produced in most service industries, introduces the reader to various definitions of "emotional care" given by providers to patients and of "emotional support" that caregivers themselves need in order to prevent long term exhaustion and ensure their well being. She underscores the need for research and practice developments to find better and more effective ways to "take care of the carers," both within health care delivery systems and within society in general.

In chapter 6, Gilbert Pinard reviews research on intense negative emotions, often experienced at clinical levels, that are associated with surgery and severe illnesses. He discusses how people's emotions impact on various aspects of health care, such as the rapidity with which they consult, the ease with which they speak of symptoms, their adherence to treatment regimens, their satisfaction with their interactions with the health care system, and how they experience their disorders. For instance, research shows that the intensity with which a patient experiences anxiety and fear at the onset of certain illnesses like a heart attack may cause that person to delay seeking treatment, even when that person knows that the optimal efficacy of care is related to earlier intervention. Depression also has a significant impact on health and the health care system. The odds that a person suffering from a myocardial infarction will die from the condition are more than tripled if a history of major depression is present. The cost of care increases by more than 40 per cent if a patient who has coronary heart disease also suffers from depression. The author also reflects on how the restructuring and downsizing of the health care system and the trend of "outsourcing care to the family" affects caregivers, be they professionals or patients' family members.

In chapter 7, Laurette Dubé focuses on emotions as they are experienced at below clinical levels in everyday contexts, such as during episodes of illness and care. Positive and negative emotions are feeling states that signal the occurrence of events that are personally relevant, motivating those who feel them to act in certain manners and others to respond to them in specific ways. She suggests that the emotions patients experience in the course of the delivery of care offer cues that providers may use to help design and deliver more effective health interventions. She reviews basic approaches to the measurement of everyday emotions and proposes that one can "engineer" (i.e., mindfully design and manage) caregivers' responses to patients' emotions in order to create the most positive patient and provider outcomes. Presenting empirical findings from research conducted in various contexts, including the health domain, the author argues that an evidence-based approach to testing alternative provider responses to patient emotions is a challenging endeavour because of the subjective nature of emotional experience but that it is feasible and necessary to understanding interventions directed at the human facets of care.

THE SCIENCE OF CARE: FOCUS ON INTERPERSONAL PROCESSES

Section 3 discusses various dimensions of the interpersonal processes involved in the delivery of health care. The bulk of the research in this area has consisted primarily of microscopic analyses of verbal and non-verbal exchanges in patient-physician encounters and the link between these exchanges and care outcomes.

Debra L. Roter, the author of chapter 8, is a pioneer in this line of research. Her work has demonstrated that the quality of this interactive process is critical to the establishment of a sound therapeutic relationship, with more positive outcomes being generally tied to patient-centred interactions that are based on responsiveness, facilitativeness, informativeness, and participation. In this chapter, she reports findings concerning gender differences that indicate that female physicians are more inclined to adopt a patient-centred communication style than are their male colleagues. Women physicians are more responsive to patients' emotions: They use more empathy, self-disclosure, reassurance, and concern; they are more likely to facilitate verbal exchanges by being less verbally dominant and by eliciting more information; they provide more information, especially in the psychosocial domain, and they use more partnership statements.

In chapter 9, Heather Boon further explores the patient-physician relationship by presenting a comprehensive review of the literature on the effects that different physician communication styles have on patient outcomes. Reports indicate that good communication skills on the part of the physician include expressing concern, showing support, and empathizing. These skills result in higher levels of patient satisfaction, increased adherence to treatment, and better patient health outcomes. More specifically, patient adherence to treatment has been shown to be higher when the provider uses communication styles that favour the exchange of information, such as ensuring the patient understands, or that make use of "facilitating comments," such as ensuring the patient plays an active role in the interaction. She discusses the reliance on practitioners of complementary medicine (e.g., naturopaths) by close to 50 per cent of the population in Canada and in the US and then compares patient-provider communication in conventional (patient-family physician) and complementary (patient-naturopathic practitioner) contexts. Preliminary results from a small-scale pilot study suggest that even though the duration of the visit is much shorter in the conventional compared to the complementary context, conventional and complementary practitioners may not necessarily vary in their degree of patient-centredness. In both cases, good providers were identified by patients as those who listened to patients, encouraged questions, and made patients feel cared for. The author underscores the need for further empirical investigation of the similarities and differences in patient-provider interactions in the two contexts.

In chapter 10, Krista K. Trobst pursues the discussion on patient-provider relationships by proposing a reconceptualization of professional health services that emphasizes an interpersonal social-support context. Even though social-support and patient-provider relationships have attracted attention from researchers at about the same time, there has been little cross-fertilization between the two lines of research. In bringing together these areas of study, she offers a more sophisticated conceptualization and measurement of the "human" aspects of care in terms of the specific social support strategies they entail. A model is presented, the Support Actions Scale Circumplex (SAS-C), that permits the assessment of a broad range of social support behaviours. In contrast to other models and measures of social support, the SAS-C model is multifaceted. It surveys not only the prototypically warm and accepting actions one could provide in a support situation, but also several forms of more confrontive, dismissive, or avoidant actions. In other words, this model allows for the capture of both the good and the bad in support exchanges. Furthermore, the SAS-C model captures a much broader array of social support behaviours than is typically assessed with other commonly employed measures. The author presents the reader with an illustration of how this model can be used to elucidate patient-provider relationships.

CHALLENGES IN INTEGRATING THE ART AND SCIENCE OF CARE INTO HEALTH RESEARCH AND PRACTICE

Attempts at a full and systematic integration of the art and science of emotions and interpersonal behaviour with health research and practice have remained relatively scarce. Emotions are complex and highly idiographic phenomena, and their investigation in a day-to-day context requires conceptual and methodological approaches that were unavailable until recently. Difficulties when studying the interpersonal dimensions of health care lie in the interactive, dynamic nature of patient-provider interactions. Further challenges are presented by the complex systems and by the various professional practices that, in modern times, have become unavoidable intermediaries between the patient and the doctor, potentially impeding or facilitating any intervention aimed at a better integration of the human aspects of care into everyday health practice.

In the last section, contributors offer examples of conceptual, analytical, and innovative approaches to action research that may help alleviate these difficulties and better equip care givers to face challenges in understanding and pursing better practices in the art of care.

In chapter 11, D.S. Moskowitz demonstrates how concepts from basic social sciences disciplines like psychology can foster a better theoretical understanding of the emotional and interpersonal aspects of health care and of their impact on clinical outcomes. Using a broad conceptual framework of interpersonal behaviours, the Interpersonal Circumplex model, she examines how affect and behaviour fluctuate, their mutual impact on each other, and how knowing about these dynamics may be useful in increasing motivation in patients to adopt behaviours that would help them maintain or better their health. According to the Interpersonal Circumplex model, the behaviours people adopt when interacting with others vary along two dimensions. The first dimension of interpersonal interaction refers to actions that connect the individual to others (referred to as communal or affiliative behaviours), while a second fundamental dimension refers to attempts to assert the self and raise or maintain the individual's status relative to the other (referred to as agentic, power, and status behaviours). The author presents results from field studies illustrating these dimensions and suggests how the model could prove useful in improving patient and health care provider relationships. It is argued that health care workers should (1) try to promote communal behaviours in patients that serve to create an affiliative bond between the health care worker and the patient, and (2) encourage patients to give information, make suggestions, and set goals – behaviours that maintain and increase the patient's sense of agency. Improving the affiliative bond and the patient's sense of influence on the interactions should contribute to an improved collaborative alliance between the patient and the health care provider.

In chapter 12, Lawrence R. Levy, Richard W.J. Neufeld, and Weiguang Yao present analytical difficulties and challenges. The authors reflect on how many of the human aspects of care discussed in this volume, such as emotions, patient-provider relationships, and social support, could benefit from being investigated using a dynamic systems approach. Defined as the study of the manner in which a system changes over time, non-linear dynamical system theory (also known as chaos theory) is a powerful tool that can mathematically quantify such concepts as temporality, multidimensionality, and interdependence. This approach can model short-term predictability, which can then aid the researcher in speculating about the future behaviour of the system. For instance, the dynamic systems methodology could be utilized to better understand the complex, multifaceted, multidimensional, and interrelational aspects of emotions in the provision of health care. The richness of this approach stems from its capacity to simulate, via computer, how various dimensions interact with one another, how these interactions unfold temporally, and how the system eventually reaches an optimal state of stability. Examples are presented of research contexts that have successfully used the dynamic systems approach.

In chapter 13, Terrence Montague addresses two important challenges to integrating the human aspects of care with health research and practice. The first challenge is to identify efficacious interventions through rigorous empirical testing of the impact of alternative care provision strategies on the outcomes of care. He underscores the need to understand the value systems of the contexts in which empirical assessments occur. The second challenge is to identify gaps that impede the implementation and use of efficacious interventions such that the best care is not always provided or is not provided to its full potential. The author uses prescription drug medications as an example of the "care gap" – that is, the gap between best care, as defined by proven efficacious therapy, and usual care, or the actual care being provided to the population at risk. This gap is influenced by several factors, including poor diagnosis or poor prescription by physicians, unwillingness or inability of patients to follow prescription recommendations, and restricted access to health care. Any one of these gaps or their combination will result in suboptimal outcomes in the population. The author reports on an innovative, interdisciplinary, action-oriented research undertaking by the Clinical Quality Improvement Network (CQIN), a group of physicians, pharmacists, nurses, and other health care workers and researchers concerned about the care gap. On the basis of an empirical assessment, the CQIN team has developed strategies for closing the care gap by addressing a set of underlying causes. The strategy involves creating a broad-based, grass-roots partnership whose members measure and analyze practices and outcomes. Investigated through various studies conducted in University of Alberta hospitals, this strategy has successfully increased the utilization of proven drugs and decreased the reliance on non-proven drugs in the management of heart attack patients, while decreasing in-hospital patient mortality.

CONCLUSION

The concepts, methods, and findings gathered in this book form a limited-scope inventory of the "science of care," whose development, we argue, should be fostered to help patients and care givers more effectively face the challenges of managing health as part of everyday life. The issue of managing health care in everyday life is particularly timely given the prevalence of chronic diseases and their projected increase with the aging of the population.

This compilation is intended for scholars in basic disciplines interested in emotions and interpersonal processes and in the role they play in health. It is also intended for health care researchers and providers interested in the integration of these dimensions into their own research endeavours and professional practices. We hope this book will stimulate further thinking about the "art of care," giving rise to new models, new practices, and new strategies at the dyadic, team, and institutional levels. These chapters may stimulate research projects and field actions concerned with the emotional and interpersonal aspects of care that combine sophisticated theoretical models, rigorous empirical testing of the efficacy of interventions, and ecological validity for the context, while contributing to the design and management of more effective health care interventions, including pertinent regulations and public policies.

2

Measuring the Quality
of the Primary Care Relationship

DANA GELB SAFRAN

From the earliest definitions of the term primary care to the most recent, all have stressed that primary care is predicated on a sustained relationship between patients and the clinician(s) who care for them (Institute of Medicine 1978, 1996; Millis 1966; Alpert and Charney 1973; Starfield 1992). Similarly, a distinctive feature of primary care is its focus on the whole person in the context both of patients' personal and medical histories and of their life circumstances, rather than a focus on particular diseases, organs, or systems. And finally, the primary physician has a distinctive role with respect to integrating the care that patients receive within and outside of the primary care setting.

This unique role was aptly summarized by a physician whom I interviewed as part of a 1994 study on defining primary care: "Other men and women are responsible for different parts and pieces and different areas, but there must be, there has to be, there should be one person responsible for the whole picture ... [w]ho has the ability cognitively and emotionally, to put it all together and to put the different recommendations into the context of that patient's life" (Safran 1994a, 4).

In this chapter, I present a review of the extensive research I have conducted since 1990 on quality in primary care. This work has been done with numerous collaborators (see references) whose significant contributions I want to acknowledge. My particularly deep appreciation goes to William H. Rogers, whose partnership since the inception of this work has been critical to our shared accomplishments, and to Alvin R. Tarlov, MD, and John E. Ware, PhD, whose insights during initial stages of this research inspired me to see it through.

The Institute of Medicine Committee on the Future of Primary Care posited the following definition: "Primary care is the provision of integrated, accessible health care services by clinicians who are accountable for addressing a large majority of personal health care needs, developing a sustained partnership with patients, and practicing in the context of family and the community" (Institute of Medicine 1996, 31). Like earlier definitions of primary care, this definition posits primary care to be defined in accordance with a set of distinctive and necessary characteristics of the care itself, rather than by the characteristics of the clinicians who provide the care or by the settings in which it is provided.

The Primary Care Assessment Survey (PCAS) (Safran, Kosinski, Tarlov, Rogers, Taira, Lieberman, et al. 1998d) is a fifty-one-item, validated, patient-completed questionnaire designed to measure each of the essential features of primary care posited by the Institute of Medicine (IOM) definition and others (Institute of Medicine 1978). The survey is intended for performance measurement and quality improvement at the individual physician, group practice, health plan, or delivery system level. The PCAS provides an assessment of seven domains of primary care through eleven summary scales, as follows: access (financial and organizational), continuity (relationship duration, visit-based), comprehensiveness ("whole-person" knowledge of the patient, preventive counselling), integration of care, quality of the clinical interaction (clinician-patient communication, thoroughness of physical examinations), interpersonal treatment, and trust. Figure 1 illustrates the seven domains and eleven summary scales that comprise the PCAS.

All concepts in the PCAS are measured in the context of a specific clinician-patient primary care relationship and reference the entirety of that relationship (i.e., they are not visit-specific). This is consistent with the IOM definition and others, which emphasize that primary care is founded on sustained clinician-patient relationships (Institute of Medicine 1978, 1996; Millis 1966; Alpert and Charney 1973; Starfield 1992). A single screener item is used to determine whether the respondent has an established relationship with a primary clinician (or team of primary clinicians). Only those indicating such a relationship complete the remaining PCAS items. The PCAS was developed for use in a general adult population, though a paediatric version of the questionnaire has been developed.

This chapter begins by providing an overview of the rationale for using patient-provided information to assess primary care performance. It then describes the development of the Primary Care Assessment Survey and summarizes its measurement properties. Finally, it describes some recent applications of the PCAS in research to identify the organizational and individual factors that influence primary care performance and to determine the extent to which primary care performance predicts important outcomes of care.

Figure 1
Essential attributes of primary care measured
by the Primary Care Assessment Survey (PCAS)

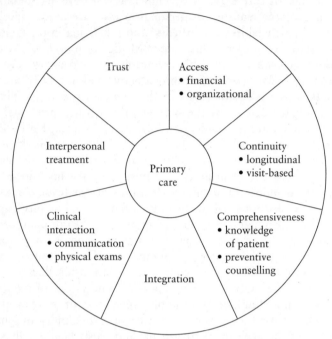

Source: Copyright 2000 Lawrence Erlbaum Associates, Inc. Reprinted, with permission of the
publisher, from A. Murray and D.G. Safran, "The Primary Care Assessment Survey: A tool for
measuring, monitoring, and improving primary care," in M.E. Maruish, ed., *Handbook of
Psychological Assessment* (Mahwah, NJ: Lawrence Erlbaum Associates, Inc., 2000), 624.

WHY USE PATIENT-PROVIDED INFORMATION TO ASSESS CARE?

With the increasing emphasis on quality assessment and continuous
quality improvement, patients have emerged as an important source of
information about health care. Patient-provided information has
important strengths and limitations that must be taken into account in
designing a quality assessment initiative and in interpreting data from it.

With respect to primary care quality assessment, there are four
salient strengths of patient-provided information. First, patient-provided
data are generally less expensive to obtain than comparable data from
other sources (e.g., health plan administration, physician, other health
staff) (Davies and Ware 1988). Second, since no documentation of

performance on many defining elements of primary care currently exists in administrative data collection systems, information must be obtained either by observation of the primary care process (which would be both costly and intrusive) or from its participants (i.e., patient, clinician, health plan administration). In the latter case, patients have less motivation to distort ratings and reports than might sources who are directly accountable for care.

Third, the reliability and validity of patient-provided information concerning important elements of care, including access, continuity, and interpersonal treatment, have been extensively documented (Ware, Snyder, Wright, and Part 1976; Davies, Ware, Brook, Peterson, and Newhouse 1986; United States States Congress Office of Technology Assessment 1988; Gerbert and Hargreaves 1986; Brown and Adams 1992; Aday and Anderssen 1975; Aday, Anderssen, and Flemming 1980; Sox, Margulies, and Sox 1981). For example, studies have shown patients' assessments of the interpersonal aspects of care accord with assessments made by trained observers of the medical encounter (Stiles, Putnam, James, and Wolf 1979; Di Matteo and Hays 1980). Moreover, patients' reports about specific occurrences related to their care (e.g., whether a test was performed, a treatment recommended, a particular clinician seen) have proven highly accurate – in fact, as accurate as physicians' reports about these occurrences (Davies 1988; Gerbret and Hargreaves 1986; Brown and Adams 1992; Montano and Phillips 1995; Lewis 1988; Zapka, Palmer, Hargreaves, Nerenz, Frazier, and Warner 1995).

Patient assessments of technical quality of care are the sole exception and represent an important limitation of patient-provided information concerning health care. With respect to the technical quality of care, evidence concerning the reliability and validity of patient-provided information is mixed. On the one hand, patients have been shown to appropriately discriminate between encounters judged by physicians to differ in the quality of medical history solicitation and physical examination (Davies 1988; Ware 1978a). On the other hand, there is evidence that patients' ratings of technical quality of care are influenced by the *amount* of care received (i.e., more is better) and by the degree of interpersonal treatment (Ware et al. 1976; Davies et al. 1986; United States Congress Office of Technology Assessment 1988; Gerbert and Hargreaves 1986; Sox et al. 1981). For this reason, as noted above, the PCAS conducts only a limited assessment related to technical quality, using a questionnaire item concerning thoroughness of physical examination for which the reliability and validity of patient-provided information has been established.

A fourth advantage of patient-provided information about care is that patients' assessments of their care have been linked to important outcomes of care, including patients' adherence to medical advice, utilization of available care, other care-seeking behaviour (including disenrolment from a physician's practice or a health plan), and health outcomes (Ware and Davies 1983; Murphy, Chang, Montgomery, Rogers, and Safran 2001; Greenfield, Kaplan, and Ware 1985; Greenfield, Kaplan, Ware, Yano, and Franck 1988; Safran, Taira, Rogers, Kosinski, Ware, and Tarlov, 1998b). Studies of adherence, for example, have demonstrated that it is positively associated with: (1) effective clinician-patient communication (Di Matteo 1994; Di Matteo, Sherbourne, Hays, Ordway, Kravitz, McGlynn, et al. 1993; Smith, Polis, and Hadac 1981); (2) continuity in the clinician-patient relationship (Charney, Bynum, Eldridge, Franck, MacWhinney, McNabb, et al. 1967; Becker, Drachman, and Kirscht 1974); and (3) humane interpersonal treatment (Eraker, Kirscht, and Becker 1984; Francis, Korsch, and Morris 1969). More recently, a study using the PCAS reaffirmed the relationship of each of these factors to adherence but suggested that patients' trust in their physicians and physicians' comprehensive knowledge of their patients supersede all other factors in the strength of their relationship to adherence (Safran et al. 1998b). With all other factors remaining constant, adherence rates were nearly three times higher in primary care relationships characterized by very high levels of trust and "whole-person" knowledge than in those with very low levels. PCAS scales were also significant predictors of patients' satisfaction with their physicians and of patients' self-reported changes in overall health during the previous four years.

In summary, patient-provided information about care represents considerably more than a simplistic marker of patient satisfaction. A substantial body of empirical research demonstrates that patients can reliably report about and evaluate numerous essential aspects of health care. Moreover, in addition to providing an accurate portrayal of the patient's health care experience, patient-provided information about care predicts important outcomes of care. In this way, patients' assessments of health care are distinguished from assessments of other services that people are asked to evaluate. Unlike an airline passenger, for example, whose assessment of the service received on a flight has no bearing on the probability that his plane will crash, a patient's assessment of the care he or she receives is directly linked to whether his or her metaphorical "plane" will crash. The link is due to patients' behaviours being influenced by patients' experiences in the care setting, particularly by the quality of relationships established with clinicians.

DEVELOPMENT AND TESTING OF THE PRIMARY CARE ASSESSMENT SURVEY

The item-content and descriptive information concerning the eleven PCAS scales is summarized in Table 1. Two stages of analysis were used to evaluate the measurement properties of the PCAS scales (Safran et al. 1998d). In the first stage, five scaling assumptions were tested that must be satisfied to ensure the appropriate application of Likert's summated rating scales. This stage of analysis was applicable only to the seven scales comprised of multiple evaluative items, those for which Likert's scaling method was used. In the second stage, all eleven scales were assessed for data completeness, score distribution characteristics, and interscale correlations. All analyses were conducted in the combined population and replicated in sixteen population subgroups defined according to age, sex, race, years of education, household income, and health status. Subgroup analyses were conducted to ensure that measures were applied adequately across varied segments of the population. The results suggest that the PCAS has excellent measurement properties and that it performs consistently well across varied sectors of the population. Details of the methods and results of these analyses are summarized in the following sections

Tests of Likert Scaling Assumptions

Seven PCAS scales are scored based on Likert's use of summated rating scales. The Likert method assumes that item responses from the separate scales can be combined without standardization or weighting (Likert 1932). Five scaling assumptions must be met for this form of item aggregation to be appropriate. These assumptions are: (1) that each item correlates substantially with its hypothesized scale (item-convergent validity); (2) that items within a scale correlate more substantially with their hypothesized scale than with any other scale (item-discriminant validity); (3) that items within a scale have approximately equal means and variances (equal item variance); (4) that all items in a scale contribute approximately the same proportion of information about the underlying concept (equal item-scale correlations); and (5) that scores be reproducible and reliable (score reliability). The Revised Multitrait Attribute Program, a microcomputer software application for psychometric testing, was used to test these five assumptions in the seven multi-item evaluative scales (Hays and Hayshi 1990)

Results from tests of the five scaling assumptions are summarized in Table 2 and described in the sections that follow. For a more complete report about these results, see Safran et al. 1998d.

Item-convergent validity. This scaling assumption is evaluated on the basis of item-scale correlations (i.e., each item correlated with its hypothesized scale). Item-convergent validity is supported if, after correcting for overlap (i.e., estimating the item-scale correlation with the

Table 1
Descriptive characteristics and content of the Primary Care Assessment Survey (PCAS) scales

Scale	No. of items[a]	Response format	Item content
Financial access	2	Rating	Assessment of the amount of money patient pays for doctor visits and for prescribed treatments
Organizational access	6	Rating	Ability to get through to the physician's office by telephone, to get a medical appointment when sick, and to obtain information by telephone; punctuality of appointments, convenience of office location, and convenience of office hours
Longitudinal continuity	1	Report	Duration of patient's relationship with primary physician
Visit-based continuity	2	Report	How often patient sees primary physician (not an assistant or partner) for routine check-ups and for appointments when sick
Contextual knowledge of the patient	5	Rating	Primary physician's knowledge of patient's medical history, responsibilities at work, home, or school, principal health concerns, and values and beliefs
Preventive counselling	7	Report	Whether primary physician has discussed the following with patient: smoking, alcohol use, seat belt use, diet, exercise, stress, safe sex[b]
Integration	6	Rating	Assessment of primary physician's role in coordinating and synthesizing care received from specialists and/or while patient was hospitalized
Communication	6	Rating	Thoroughness of primary physician's questions about symptoms, attention to what patient says, clarity of explanations and instructions, and advice and help in making decisions about care
Physical exams	1	Rating	Thoroughness of primary physician's physical examinations of patient
Interpersonal treatment	5	Rating	Primary physician's patience, friendliness, caring, respect, and time spent with patient
Trust	8	Rating	Assessment of primary physician's integrity, competence, and role as the patient's agent

Source: Copyright 1998 Lippincott Williams & Wilkins. Reprinted, with permission of the publisher, from D.G. Safran, M. Kosinski, A.R. Tarlov, W.H. Rogers, D.A. Taira, N. Lieberman, et al., 1998d, "The Primary Care Assessment Survey: Tests of data quality and measurement performance," *Medical Care* 36 (1998): 730.

[a] The PCAS includes fifty-nine items: forty-nine items listed here and two screener items (not listed). Only patients who respond affirmatively to the first screener item (indicate having a primary clinician or team of primary clinicians) complete the remaining PCAS items. Only patients who report having received specialty and/or hospital care (second screener item) complete the items in the "integration" scale.

[b] These topics correspond to seven behavioural risks that the U.S. Preventive Services Task Force (1989) recommends every primary physician address with every adult patient, regardless of age, sex, race, ethnicity, or other personal characteristics. Attention to preventive care has been suggested as a useful proxy for comprehensiveness of care given the difficulty of otherwise monitoring and quantifying all services and treatments provided.

Table 2
Tests of Likert scaling assumptions, total analytic sample

Scale	Range of item-scale correlations[a] (assumptions #1, #4)	Item scaling tests (assumption #2)		Measures of equal item variance (assumption #3)		Cronbach's alpha (assumption #5)
		Success/Total[b]	Scaling success rate (%)	Scott's homogeneity[c]	Intraclass correlation[d]	
Financial access	0.67 – 0.67	22/22	100.0	0.67	0.67	.81
Organizational access	0.42 – 0.69	66/66	100.0	0.46	0.46	.84
Contextual knowledge of patient	0.63 – 0.85	55/55	100.0	0.69	0.69	.92
Integration	0.63 – 0.86	66/66	100.0	0.66	0.67	.92
Communication	0.68 – 0.90	66/66	100.0	0.77	0.78	.95
Interpersonal treatment	0.78 – 0.92	55/55	100.0	0.81	0.81	.95
Trust	0.49 – 0.73	87/88	98.9	0.43	0.44	.86

Source: Copyright 1998 Lippincott Williams & Wilkins. Reprinted, with permission of the publisher, from D.G. Safran, M. Kosinski, A.R. Tarlov, W.H. Rogers, D.A. Taira, N. Lieberman, et al., 1998d, "The Primary Care Assessment Survey: Tests of data quality and measurement performance," *Medical Care* 36 (1998): 733.

[a] Range of correlations between items and their hypothesized (parent) scale correlated for overlap

[b] Each item in each scale is tested to assure that its correlation with the hypothesized (parent) scale is substantially greater than its correlation with any other (non-parent) scale. In this ratio, the denominator represents the total number of item-scale correlations tested (i.e., all items in the scale tested against all scales). The numerator represents the number of these correlations for which the items in the scale correlate significantly higher with the parent scale than with any other scale. The scaling success rate translates this ratio into a percentage; 100 per cent represents perfect scaling success.

[c] Average interitem correlation for standardized items (mean = 0; sd = 1)

[d] Average of interitem correlations

item removed from its hypothesized scale) (Howard and Forehand 1962) an item correlates 0.30 or greater with its hypothesized scale. All PCAS item-scale correlations (corrected for overlap) well exceeded the accepted minimum (0.30) in the combined population and all population subgroups (Safran et al. 1998d). The vast majority of item-scale correlations (86.5 per cent) were greater than 0.60 (Table 2).

Item-discriminant validity. This scaling assumption was tested by contrasting each item's correlation to its hypothesized scale (corrected for overlap) with its correlation to all other scales. Steiger's t-test for dependent correlations was used to test the significance of the difference between two item-scale correlations (Steiger 1980). Scaling success is expressed as a percentage and indicates how often items within a scale correlate significantly more with their hypothesized scale than with any other scale. One hundred per cent represents perfect scaling success.

Six of the seven multi-item scales achieved 100 per cent scaling success, indicating that all items in these scales correlated substantially higher with their hypothesized scale than with any other scale (Table 2). The trust scale achieved 98.9 per cent scaling success because of one item that correlated equally with another scale (contextual knowledge). The item was retained because its inclusion in the trust scale was supported by other theoretical and psychometric standards (Safran et al. 1998d). Scaling success rates were similarly high in each of the sixteen population subgroups.

Equal item variance. The assumption of equal item variance was tested through a combination of visual inspection of item means and variances and through the use of two statistics computed by multitrait analysis: Scott's coefficient of homogeneity (Scott 1968) and the intraclass correlation coefficient. If the intraclass correlation coefficient is equal to Scott's homogeneity ratio, items in a scale are judged to have approximately equal variances. Equal item variance was well supported for all multi-item scales. Item means differed by less than four-tenths of a point, and item standard deviations differed by less than three-tenths of a point (Safran et al. 1998d). The intraclass correlation coefficient and Scott's homogeneity ratio were approximately equal to one another for each scale, providing further indication of equal item variance (Table 2).

Equal item-scale correlations. The assumption of equal item-scale correlations is tested by computing item-scale correlations (corrected for overlap) for each scale and by inspecting the range of correlations obtained for all items in a scale. A narrow range indicates support for equal item-scale correlations. All PCAS scales demonstrated a relatively narrow range of item-scale correlations (Table 2). Two scales (organizational access and trust) had wider ranges because of a single item in each that was a low outlier in correlation to its parent scale. These items were retained because they were supported as important items by other psychometric indicators.

Score reliability. Two measures of reliability were used to test this fifth scaling assumption: (1) Cronbach's alpha coefficient and (2) test-retest reliability. Cronbach's alpha coefficient (Cronbach 1970) measures the internal consistency reliability of a scale (i.e., the degree to which the items that comprise a scale measure the same underlying concept). An alpha coefficient of at least 0.70 is recommended for group-level comparisons (Nunnelly and Berstein 1994). Data for test-retest analyses were obtained by administering a second (abbreviated) survey to a random sample of respondents (n = 500). The second survey contained eight PCAS items and nine supplementary items (including an item to assess the number of medical visits made since completing the initial survey). Test-retest reliability was assessed with a Pearson correlation coefficient for each PCAS item administered in both surveys. The sensitivity of the results to the time interval between test and retest, and to the occurrence of additional visits between test and retest, was assessed.

All scales exceeded the established standard for internal consistency reliability for group-level comparisons (Cronbach's alpha of 0.70) (Cronbach 1970). Alpha coefficients ranged from 0.81 (financial access) to 0.95 (communication, interpersonal treatment) in the combined population (Table 2) and were similarly high across all population subgroups. Table 3 presents estimates of test-retest reliability for the eight PCAS items administered twice to a subset of respondents. Overall, item-level correlations were higher among patients with no intervening visits than among patients with at least one intervening visit (median correlation 0.67 and 0.65, respectively) and higher among patients with shorter time intervals between surveys than among those with longer intervals (medical correlation 0.65 and 0.62, respectively).

Tests of Measurement Performance on All Scales

Three features of measurement performance were assessed for all eleven PCAS scales: data completeness, score distribution characteristics, and interscale correlations. Completeness of data is an important

Table 3

Item-level test-retest correlations for eight PCAS items by number of intervening medical visits

Rating items	Intervening visits		Length of retest interval	
	None (n = 111)	One or more (n = 152)	Shorter than median (5–13 weeks) (n = 165)	Median (14 weeks) (n = 109)
Appointment wait (ORG1)	0.70	0.52	0.64	0.48
Office wait (ORG2)	0.65	0.66	0.66	0.65
Doctor's office location (ORG5)	0.61	0.57	0.63	0.48
Hours open (ORG6)	0.58	0.57	0.55	0.62
Amount patient pays for visit (FIN1)	0.58	0.72	0.72	0.60
Amount patient pays for medication (FIN2)	0.68	0.71	0.68	0.72
See regular doctor for routine care (CONTV1)	0.72	0.64	0.71	0.52
See regular doctor when sick (CONTV2)	0.74	0.75	0.80	0.60
Median (all items)	0.67	0.65	0.65	0.62

Source: Copyright 2000 Lawrence Erlbaum Associates, Inc. Reprinted, with permission of the publisher, from A. Murray and D.G. Safran, "The Primary Care Assessment Survey: A tool for measuring, monitoring, and improving primary care," in M.E. Maruish, ed., *Handbook of Psychological Assessment* (Mahwah, NJ: Lawrence Erlbaum Associates, Inc, 2000), 633.

[a] The median and maximum time interval between receipt of test and retest surveys was fourteen weeks. The fourteen-week interval occurred among those who responded most promptly to the initial survey.

criterion by which to evaluate a scale and/or survey in that substantial amounts of missing data may suggest that items are difficult to understand or that respondents find them objectionable. Score distribution characteristics are important in that, for a scale to yield meaningful information, either as a dependent or independent variable, a sufficient variability of responses must be obtained. Indicators of score distributions include skewness, range, and percentage of respondents with the lowest possible score (floor) and highest possible score (ceiling). Finally, comparing interscale correlations with scale score reliability (alpha coefficients) provides a means of assessing the uniqueness of the concepts measured by each scale. That is, to the extent that a scale's alpha coefficient exceeds its correlation with any other scale, there is evidence of unique reliable variance measured by that scale. Establishing evidence for the distinctiveness of each scale is important for the interpretability of scale scores and, in practical terms, helps justify the value of scaling and reporting each separately.

Data completeness. Completeness of data was assessed by computing the percentage of item levels missing data for each of the items used in scoring the eleven PCAS scales. In addition, for each scale, we computed the percentage of respondents (combined population and sixteen subgroups) for which a score was computable (i.e., the individual responded to at least half of the scale items). Missing value rates for all PCAS items were low, ranging from 0.0% to 4.2%. The percentage of the population with computable scores ranged from 98.3 to 99.9 in both the combined population and the subgroups. The high data completeness rates indicate the acceptability to respondents of the survey content and length.

Score distribution characteristics. All evaluative scales were negatively skewed, indicating distributions with more positive ratings of primary care. The full range of possible scores (0 to 100) was observed for all scales except one (trust). This suggests that the full range of response choices offered within each scale's constituent items was meaningful to respondents. The percentage of respondents scoring at the floor and ceiling was acceptably low for all multi-item evaluative scales. The most substantial ceiling effects occurred for the report-format continuity scales and for the single-item evaluative measure (thoroughness of physical exams), due to the smaller number of response categories (levels) in these measures (Safran et al. 1998d).

Interscale correlations. In all cases, Cronbach's alpha coefficients for the PCAS scale substantially exceed the scale's correlation with all other scales. Approximately half of the scale-scale correlations (26 of 55) were less than 0.36. The highest scale-scale correlation occurred between communication and interpersonal treatment (0.86), although the alpha coefficients for both were substantially higher (0.95). The findings support the value and importance of separately measuring and interpreting the concepts reflected in the eleven PCAS scales.

SUMMARY OF A LONGITUDINAL APPLICATION OF THE PCAS

From 1996 through 1999, we applied the Primary Care Assessment Survey in a longitudinal observational study of insured adults in Massachusetts. The study aimed to identify the organizational and individual characteristics that influence primary care performance and to learn how primary care performance predicts important outcomes of care. The study was conducted with funding from the Agency for Health Care Policy and Research (AHCPR ROI HS-08841) and the Robert Wood Johnson Foundation (RWJF Grant #35321). The study methods and results are summarized here.

Study Population

The sample frame for the study consisted of all active adult employees (eighteen years and older) of the Commonwealth of Massachusetts in 1995 who subscribed to one of twelve health plans offered to state workers. Initial data for the study were obtained between January and April 1996 using a four-step protocol for mail surveys (Dillman 1978) supplemented by telephone follow-up to a sample of non-respondents. A 69 per cent response rate was achieved, with 6,810 responses obtained by mail and 394 obtained by telephone. The mean age of the respondent population was forty-eight (range: nineteen to eighty-eight). Just over half of the respondents (55 per cent) were female, and the vast majority were white (87 per cent), with more than a high-school education (70 per cent). These population characteristics are reflective of employed adults nationally except that a larger proportion of state employees are college educated and in older age groups (forty-five years and older). Physical and mental health summary scores, derived from the Short-Form 12-Item Health Survey (SF-12), were approximately the same as those of the general US adult population and somewhat lower than those of employed adults nationally (Ware, Kosinski, and Keller 1996a; Ware, Snow, Kosinski, and Gandek 1993).

Ninety-one per cent of patients reported having a primary physician. Of these, 87 per cent identified a generalist physician, 2 per cent identified an obstetrician/gynecologist, and 11 per cent identified a physician in another specialty or medical subspecialty. These findings are consistent with those from national studies that have assessed the percentage of Americans who report having a primary physician and the extent of specialist physicians' involvement in this role (Aiken, Lewis, Craig, Mendenhall, Blendon, and Rogers 1979; Smith and Buesching 1986; Spiegel, Rubenstein, Scott, and Brook 1983; Falik and Scott 1996).

Linking Primary Care Performance to Important Outcomes of Care

In the initial cross-sectional survey, sustained primary care partnerships characterized by bonds of trust and physician's "whole-person" knowledge of patients were observed to be the leading correlates of three important outcomes of care: adherence, satisfaction, and improved health status (Safran et al. 1998b). The results were noteworthy in the context of changes to the US's health care system that many patients, clinicians, medical educators, and policy makers have speculated threaten the therapeutic alliance between doctor and patient (Mechanic 1996; Scott, Aiken, Mechanic, and Moravcsik 1995; Leopold, Cooper, and Clancy 1996; Emanuel and Dubler 1995; Barr 1995; AMA Council on Ethical and Judicial Affairs 1995). The recent IOM report, along with previous definitions of primary care, assert that these attributes are essential to primary care and part of what distinguishes it from the rest of medical practice (Millis 1966; Alpert and Charney 1973; Starfield 1992; Institute of Medicine 1994). The longitudinal follow-up of the study population in 1999 allowed us to examine the causal sequences linking primary care performance at baseline (1996) and several outcomes of care. The findings are summarized next.

Primary care relationship quality as a predictor of adherence. We studied patients' adherence to their primary physicians' advice concerning four behavioral risk factors (smoking, alcohol use, exercise, and seat belt use). We used two broad categories of adherence measures: (1) patients' reported attempts to modify a risk behaviour based on their physicians' advice ("process" measure of adherence); and (2) measured change in behavioural risk factors between 1996 and 1999 among patients who were at risk in 1996 and reported having received counselling during the study period ("outcome" measure of adherence) (Safran et al. 2000a).

We found that the leading predictors of patients' reported efforts to modify a behavioural risk factor for which they have received counselling are: (1) the doctor's "whole-person" knowledge of the patient (z-score = 6.4, p < 0.001); and (2) the patient's trust in the doctor (z-score = 4.4, p < 0.001). "Outcome" adherence (i.e., measured change in behaviour) was significantly predicted by patients' baseline trust in their physicians (p = 0.05). No other relationship quality element significantly predicted measured change in risk behaviours.

Figure 2 illustrates the observed effect of trust on "process" adherence. Among patients with the lowest levels of trust in their physicians at baseline, 71 per cent attempted to modify a risk behaviour (e.g., quit smoking, lose weight) based on their physicians' advice, while 88 per cent of those with the highest levels of trust attempted behaviour change based on their physicians' advice. Similarly, among patients with the lowest levels of trust at baseline, 24 per cent *succeeded* in modifying a risk behaviour based on their physicians' advice, and 33 per cent of those with the highest levels of trust at baseline successfully modified a risk behaviour. The findings reveal the importance of relationship quality – and, in particular, patients' sense of their doctors' whole-person knowledge about them and their trust in the doctor – as determinants of adherence to medical advice. With respect to behaviour modification, relationship quality currently appears to more substantially influence *attempted* behaviour change than to influence *success* in achieving that change. Challenges remain for health professionals committed to getting their patients over the bar from attempted change to successful, sustained behaviour modification.

Figure 2
Patient trust as a predictor of adherence: Attempted behaviour change

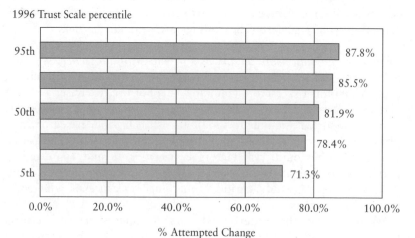

1996 Trust Scale percentile

Primary care relationship quality as a predictor of satisfaction. We examined the role of primary care relationship quality as a determinant of patients' decisions to disenrol from a health plan or from a physician's practice. Overall, 10 per cent of patients changed health plans between baseline and follow-up (1996–1999). This rate is consistent with the overall rate of plan switching among state employees from whom our sample was drawn (i.e., 3 per cent plan-switching per year). Rates of *physician* switching were considerably higher: 25 per cent of patients in the longitudinal panel changed doctors between baseline and follow-up. Most of the disenrolment from physician's practices was voluntary (20 per cent), but 5 per cent of patients had an involuntary doctor switch (i.e., the doctor died, retired, or moved a substantial distance, or the patient moved a substantial distance) (Safran, Montgomery, Chang, Murphy, and Rogers 2001b).

Relationship quality did not significantly predict patients' disenrolment from a health plan, but relationship quality was highly predictive of voluntary disenrolment from a physician's practice (Safran et al. 2001b). The role of four structural features of care (access, primary care relationship duration, visit-based continuity, and integration of care) as predictors of voluntary switching was also explored. While each of these structural features was a significant predictor of voluntary doctor switching when tested independently, these variables proved less important than relationship quality elements when tested in multivariable models. In multivariable models, a composite relationship quality factor most strongly predicted voluntary disenrolment [OR = 1.6, p < 0.001], and the two continuity scales also significantly predicted disenrolment [OR = 1.1, p < 0.05]. Access and integration did not significantly predict disenrolment in the presence of these variables. Table 4 summarizes these findings.]

The findings highlight the importance of relationship quality in determining patients' loyalty to a physician's practice. In an era marked by increasing pressure on clinicians and health care organizations to attend to such factors as market share, productivity, and efficiency, these findings point to a set of attributes that might otherwise be overlooked in the race for the bottom line. They suggest that medical practices and health plans cannot afford to ignore that the very essence of medical care delivery involves the interaction of a human being with another human being.

Primary care relationship quality as a predictor of improved health status. We examined changes in functional health status over the three-year study period and evaluated the PCAS scales as predictors of functional health outcomes. As noted above, the study population consisted

Table 4
Baseline PCAS scores as predictors of voluntary disenrolment, adjusted[a]

PCAS scale	Standardized odds ratio: model testing each scale individually [95% CI]	Standardized odds ratio: model testing scales collectively [95% CI]	Probability of disenrolment at designated percentile of pcas scale[b]				
			5th pctile	25th pctile	50th pctile	75th pctile	95th pctile
MD-patient relationship quality	1.59 [1.45, 1.74]***	1.59 [1.45, 1.74]***	37.8	25.8	19.6	15.2	12.2
Trust	1.56 [1.43, 1.71]***	–					
Interpersonal treatment	1.52 [1.39, 1.66]***	–					
MD knowledge of patient	1.51 [1.37, 1.66]***	–					
Communication	1.49 [1.36, 1.62]***	–					
Structural features of care	1.44 [1.31, 1.58]***						
Access to care	1.41 [1.27, 1.58]***	1.14 [0.98, 1.31]+	23.8	21.3	19.8	18.5	17.2
Integration		0.96 [0.81, 1.12]	–	–	–	–	–
Visit-based continuity	1.27 [1.16, 1.38]***	1.14 [1.04, 1.28]*	24.4	21.4	19.5	18.6	18.6
Relationship duration	1.29 [1.18, 1.40]***	1.16 [1.04, 1.30]**	25.3	20.5	18.3	18.3	18.3

Source: Copyright 2001 Dowden Health Media. Reprinted, with permission of the publisher, from D.G. Safran, J.E. Montgomery, H. Chang, J. Murphy, and W.H. Rogers, "Switching doctors: Predictors of voluntary disenrollment from a primary physician's practice," Journal of Family Practice 50 (2001): 134.

a Results control for patients' baseline sociodemographic profiles (age, sex, race, household income, years of education), health status (number of primary care sensitive and primary care insensitive conditions, physical functioning index, mental functioning index), and outpatient utilization (visits in the six months prior to baseline).

b Probabilities are expressed as a percentage (0–100) and are based on results of the multivariable model summarized in column 3.

+p ≤ .10, *p ≤ .05, **p ≤ .01, ***p ≤ .001

of employed adults ranging in age from nineteen to eighty-eight years at baseline (mean age = 48.6) whose health status at baseline was typical of employed adults nationally. The observed changes in health status over the three-year study period were also consistent with those expected in a population with these characteristics. The average changes in physical and mental health status (as measured by the SF-12) were each less than one point (-0.86 and +0.19 points respectively). When changes in health status were classified in categorical terms (better, same, worse), applying a methodology developed in the Medical Outcomes Study and broadly applied since that time (Ware, Bayliss, Rogers, Kosinski, and Tarlov 1996b), we found that approximately two-thirds of the study population had no significant change in their physical or mental health status. Physical health status (PCS) improved for 16 per cent and declined for 21.5 per cent. Mental health status (MCS) improved for 19 per cent and declined for 18 per cent.

Analyses relating primary care quality scales (and other variables) to health outcomes revealed no significant predictors of functional health outcomes – except age, which significantly predicted changes in physical, but not mental, health status. That is, the health of the study population did not change much over the observation period, and the changes that occurred appear to be largely associated with the natural processes of aging and not affected (positively or negatively) by the quality of primary care that patients received. In retrospect, this is a likely finding in a study of a general adult population with whom the physician and health care system have limited, sporadic involvement and for whom there is limited opportunity to substantially influence the functional health outcomes experienced over only a few years. A study involving a population of patients with substantial, specific, ongoing medical care seems an appropriate next step in an effort to evaluate whether the quality of physician-patient relationships significantly influences patients' functional health outcomes.

ORGANIZATIONAL CHARACTERISTICS AS PREDICTORS OF PRIMARY CARE PERFORMANCE

A principal objective of the study was to evaluate primary care performance using five models of managed care represented in the study: managed indemnity insurance with fees for services (FFS), point-of-service (POS), Independent Practice Association (IPA)/network-model health maintenance organization (HMO), group-model HMO, and staff-model HMO. At least four factors compelled research in this area. First, the most recent comparisons of delivery system differences in primary care performance had been based on data from the late 1970s and the

1980s (Davies et al. 1986; Safran, Tarlov, and Rogers 1994b; Luft 1980; Miller and Luft 1994; Clement, Retchin, Brown, and Stegall 1994a; Francis, Polissar, and Lorenz 1984; Murary 1988; Safran, Rogers, Tarlov, Inui, Taira, Montgomery, et al. 2000b; Rubin, Gandek, Rogers, Kosinski, McHorney, and Ware 1993; Mechanic 1975; Wolinsky 1983; Clement, Retchin, and Brown 1994b; Mechanic, Weiss, and Cleary 1983), and considerable changes in delivery systems had occurred since then – including the emergence of new forms of managed care and shifts in the populations distributed among different types of managed care. Second, advances had been made in both the definition of primary care (Institute of Medicine 1996) and in corresponding measures of primary care performance (Safran et al. 1998d), but these had not been applied in order to compare performance across different models of health insurance. Third, data characterizing primary care received by a general population of insured US adults remained unavailable as the previous data were limited to chronically ill adults. Fourth, little was known about the specific organizational structures and processes that contribute to performance differences across systems. This study aimed to fill each of these important gaps.

At baseline (1996), approximately half of the study participants (46 per cent) were enrolled in IPA/network-model HMOs, while approximately one-third were enrolled in staff- or group-model HMOs (32 per cent) and the remainder in the managed indemnity or POS plans. Thus the representation of the study population across each of five health plan types is similar to that observed among privately insured Americans nationally. The vast majority of patients (83 per cent) had been enrolled in their current health plan for three or more years.

Despite substantial health care delivery system changes in the past decade, the results of this study suggest that previously observed performance differences based on defining characteristics of primary care persist today and that substantial differences are observable for features not previously examined (i.e., physicians' knowledge of patients, communication with patients, and patients' trust) (Safran et al. 2000b; Safran et al. 1998c). Table 5 summarizes the findings. Overall, performance appears more favourable in open-model delivery systems (i.e., indemnity, POS, IPA/network-model HMO), which do not contract with physicians on an exclusive basis, than in closed-model systems (i.e., group- and staff-model HMOs). Among open-model systems, the indemnity system performed most favourably. IPA/network-model HMOs were more extensively represented here than in previous studies, and primary care performance in a point-of-service (POS) plan was evaluated for the first time. The findings suggest that these two open-model systems, which are rapidly gaining predominance in the insurance market nationwide, perform equivalently to the indemnity

Table 5
Primary care performance by health plan type, adjusted[a]

	Indemmity (n = 761)	POS (n = 579)	Network/IPA model HMO (n = 2,761)	Group model HMO (n = 934)	Staff model HMO (n = 983)
Access to care	70.6	68.0	69.2	69.2	<u>67.3</u>
Continuity					
visit-based	89.4	81.7	86.5	75.0	<u>68.9</u>
relationship duration	78.7	80.3	79.3	75.6	<u>68.9</u>
Comprehensiveness					
knowledge of the patient	58.7	55.4	56.4	56.0	<u>51.4</u>
preventive counselling	48.8	<u>44.7</u>	<u>44.6</u>	52.8	46.7
Integration	72.8	69.7	71.3	69.6	<u>65.2</u>
Clinical interaction					
physical exams	82.4	81.3	80.5	78.8	<u>75.5</u>
communication	81.1	79.8	79.6	79.2	<u>75.3</u>
Interpersonal treatment	81.2	78.8	78.6	79.2	<u>73.6</u>
Trust	78.2	76.1	76.7	75.2	<u>72.2</u>

Source: Copyright 2000 American Medical Association. Reprinted, with permission of the publisher, from D.G. Safran, W.H. Rogers, A.R. Tarlov, T.S. Inui, D.A. Taira, J.E. Montgomery, et al., "Organizational and financial characteristics of health plans: Are they related to primary care performance?" *Archives of Internal Medicine* 160 (2000): 73.

[a] Results adjust for patient sociodemographic characteristics (age, sex, race, years of education, household income), tenure in current health plan, and chronic medical conditions. For each primary care scale, **bold** type denotes the highest performing system and any system(s) statistically equivalent to it, <u>underlined</u> type denotes the lowest performing system and any system(s) statistically equivalent to it, and plain type denotes the system(s) performing at an intermediate level.

system with respect to many dimensions of primary care (Safran et al. 2000b).

To our knowledge, this is the first time that a study has differentiated between staff- and group-model HMOs, despite known differences in the nature of the contractual arrangements that the models establish for their physicians (i.e., salaried employment vs. an independent medical group contracted by the plan). The substantial differences in performance, with staff-model HMOs performing significantly less favourably with respect to all dimensions, suggests that the different contractual arrangements that the plans establish for physicians may be important.

In addition, the differing degree to which these systems rely on primary care teams, and the resulting differences in patients' continuity with their primary physician, may account for performance differences consistently reported by patients of open- vs. closed-model medical practices. Closed-model practices have historically embraced the concept of primary care teams and generally structure their care processes accordingly. For example, the appointment scheduling protocols of staff- and group-model HMOs that we have studied have almost uniformly prioritized patients' access to care over their continuity with particular clinicians. The underlying philosophy that gave rise to many of today's closed-model practices, and to the structures and processes through which they provide care, is that a clinician's technical expertise and clinical knowledge predominates in his/her ability to provide high quality care and, therefore, that care can appropriately be provided by whichever clinician from the team has the necessary level of expertise for the presenting problem (e.g., physician, nurse practitioner, other clinician) irrespective of that clinician's pre-existing knowledge about the patient.

Indeed, our study found that substantially more patients in closed-model practices reported that other clinicians play an important role in their care than did their counterparts in open-model practices (47 per cent vs. 63 per cent), yet patients' assessments of the care provided by team members was lackluster in both open- and closed-model settings. Table 6 illustrates this point, comparing patients' assessments of their primary physician with their assessments of the other clinicians on the team. Three-quarters of patients in practices that rely on teams rate the other clinicians' whole-person knowledge about them unfavourably, nearly two-thirds rate the clinicians' knowledge of their medical history unfavourably, and 55 per cent rate the clinicians' communication skills unfavourably. By comparison, patients' ratings of their primary physicians' whole-person knowledge about them were slightly better, and their primary physicians' knowledge of their medical history and communication skills was substantially better.

The data suggest that while many primary care practices – particularly closed-model settings – embrace a team approach, we are a great distance from meeting the defining criteria of primary care through teams. Most particularly, it is clear that the criteria for "sustained partnerships" between patients and their primary care clinicians and for a whole-person orientation to care are not currently being met by most team arrangements in primary care.

In summary, the observed differences in primary care performance across different models of health care delivery underscore that

Table 6
Patients' assessments of care provided by other clinicians in their primary physicians' practices vs. care provided by their primary physicians

	Other clinicians on the primary care team[a]		Primary physician		
	Excellent, very good (%)	Good, fair, poor, very poor (%)	Excellent, very good (%)	Good, fair, poor, very poor (%)	P-value[b]
Quality of care they provide	55	45	c	c	–
Coordination between them and your regular doctor	57	43	c	c	–
Their knowledge of you as a person (your values and beliefs)	24	76	29	71	.001
Their knowledge of your medical history[d]	36	64	54	46	.001
Their explanations of your health problems or treatments that you need	54	46	72	28	.001

[a] Patients who reported having a regular personal doctor were asked: Are there *other* doctors or nurses working in your regular doctor's office who play an important role in your care? Those answering affirmatively were asked a set of questions about "these *other* doctors or nurses who play an important role in your care" (results shown here).

[b] For each item, p-values compare patients' assessments of their primary care physicians with their assessments of other clinicians in the practice who play an important role in their care. Except where noted, all results are from the Massachusetts Study of Primary Care Performance, 1996 (n = 6,018), 19.

[c] This item was not asked with reference to the primary physician.

[d] Data for this item are from the Study of Choice and Quality in Senior Health Care, 1998, 23. The item was not asked in the MA study.

Source: Copyright 2003 American College of Physicians-American Society of Internal Medicine. Reprinted, with permission of the publisher, from D.G. Safran, "Defining the future of primary care: What can we learn from patients?" *Annals of Internal Medicine* 138, no. 3 (2003): 250.

differentiating among the many forms of managed care, and identifying specific organizational and financial characteristics that influence quality, are critical to furthering the value of quality assessment and the success of quality improvement. With US employers and purchasers having largely rejected traditional indemnity insurance as unaffordable, the results suggest that the current momentum toward open-model managed care plans is consistent with goals for high quality primary care but that the effects of specific organizational and financial features of care arrangements must continue to be examined.

PHYSICIAN CHARACTERISTICS
AND PRIMARY CARE PERFORMANCE

The study found few associations between primary care performance, as experienced and reported by patients, and physician age, sex, medical specialty, or work load (i.e., hours per week) (Murray, Safran, Rogers, Inui, Chang, and Montgomery 2000a). However, the relative absence of an association between these measured characteristics of physicians and primary care performance appears to tell an incomplete story. Two sets of analyses from this study suggest that physicians contribute substantially to the observed variance in primary care performance scores – even while the specific physician characteristics that account for this remain elusive.

The first set of analyses involved variance components methods, which allow determination of how the scale variance is apportioned among each of several potential "spheres of influence" – in this case, the physician, the practice site, and the health plan. For those PCAS scales that pertain directly to the doctor-patient interaction (primary care relationship duration, MD knowledge of patient, preventive counselling, integration of care, quality of communication, thoroughness of physical examinations, interpersonal treatment, and patient trust), physicians accounted for more variance in the analytic models than did health plans or practice sites combined. For structural/organizational aspects of care (organizational access, financial access, visit-based continuity), the physician's influence appeared more limited than that of plans and about equal to that of sites (Safran, Rogers, Montgomery, Murray, Chang, and Tarlov 1998a; Safran, Montgomery, Rogers, Murray, Chang, and Tarlov 1999).

The second set of analyses that highlighted physicians' substantial influence on patients' primary care experiences – as measured by the PCAS – involved an extension of the variance components models, wherein the unique identifiers denoting each primary physician, site of care, and health plan were considered in conjunction with the patients' sociodemographic profiles. In these analyses, the interaction of patients' sociodemographic profiles with the ID of their primary physicians accounted for two times more variance in the PCAS scales than did patients' sociodemographic profiles alone. The meaning of this finding is most easily understood with a concrete example – such as patient race and communication quality. In this case, the finding of a significant interaction effect between patient race and doctor ID suggests that the effect of a patient's race on the quality of doctor-patient communication depends upon *whom* the doctor is. That is, the interaction suggests that with some physicians, communication will be more favourable with minority patients (or patients in a particular minority group) and that with other physicians, it will be more favourable with non-minority patients. The substantial interaction effects between patients' sociodemographic characteristics and doctors' IDs tell us that we must look beyond any main effects associated with sociodemographics, as these appear to tell only part of the story (and a smaller part than that told by the interactions of these characteristics with the specific providers of care).

To our knowledge, this represents the first study to apply this set of hierarchical modelling techniques (including variance components and analysis of variance) in order to estimate the absolute and relative influence of physicians (as well as other domains such as practice site and health plan) on a set of quality measures. The value of this methodology in health services research, and studies of health care quality specifically, is clear – particularly when viewed in contrast to findings from analyses that employed fixed effects models. Analyses that relied on fixed effects (i.e., measured characteristics of physicians, such as age, sex, and medical specialty) yielded a very different impression of the physician's role in shaping the patient's primary care experience than is revealed through these random effects methods.

PATIENT CHARACTERISTICS
AND PRIMARY CARE PERFORMANCE

Consistent with previous research involving patient-based assessments of health care, this study found that little of the variance in primary care performance measures is accounted for by patients' sociodemographic characteristics or by their health profile. While many sociodemographic characteristics were statistically significantly related to one or more of the PCAS scales (Taira, Safran, Seto, Rogers, and Tarlov 1997b) the magnitude of these relationships was generally small (Taira, Safran, Seto, Rogers, Kosinski, Ware, et al. 1997a; Taira, Safran, Seto, Rogers, Inui, Montgomery, et al. 2001).

The study advanced beyond previous research in this area, however, by incorporating data from the US Census of Population and Housing to examine the relationship between a patient's immediate social environment and the primary care received. The results suggest that census data are a useful – perhaps even important – complement to data obtained directly from patients and that they add to the explanatory power of the models (Safran et al. 1998a; Safran et al. 1999). While we are continuing to explore the underlying basis for these effects, our hypothesis is that the block group data afford information about social class and/or socialization that is directly relevant to the patient's experience with the medical care system and that is not fully captured by a patient's age, sex, race, years of education, and household income.

The study also advanced beyond previous research in this area by applying analysis of variance methods that considered patients' sociodemographic characteristics in conjunction with a unique set of identifiers denoting their physicians, sites of care, and health plans. Together, these three sets of interaction terms accounted for an average of 12 per cent of the variance in analyses of the PCAS scales – about four times more than was explained by patients' sociodemographic profiles alone (Safran et al. 1998a). The findings suggest the value of continuing to incorporate and apply this methodology in studies of health care quality. Clearly, examining a standard set of sociodemographic indicators (as main effects) yields an incomplete impression about the relationship between patient characteristics and the quality of health care received.

MEASURING AND EXPLAINING THE CHANGE IN PRIMARY CARE RELATIONSHIP QUALITY, 1996–1999

The three-year study period (1996–1999) corresponded with a time of tremendous change in health care delivery nationally, and Massachusetts was no exception. The changes affected multiple aspects of medical practice, including the financial incentives faced by individual clinicians, the organization of medical practices, the size and configuration of health plans' physician networks, and the corporate relationships among provider organizations. The sheer quantity and momentum of change affected the environment in which health care delivery was occurring, and many of the changes had direct bearing on primary care physicians and potential bearing on their management of patient care and interactions with patients.

Using PCAS data obtained from patients in 1996 and 1999, we measured the changes in patients' experiences with their primary care physicians – including the quality of their relationships – during this three-year period (Murphy et al. 2001). Analyses were limited to patients who retained the same primary care physician throughout the study period (n = 2,383). That group of patients represented 58 per cent of the longitudinal panel and excluded patients who changed physicians and those who reported having no primary physician at one of the two observation periods. We evaluated changes in each of four elements of relationship quality (communication, interpersonal treatment, physician's knowledge of the patient, patient trust) and four structural features of care (financial access, organizational access, visit-based continuity, integration of care). Change was computed as the difference between each patient's score in 1996 and 1999, then these change scores were aggregated to determine the average change in each PCAS scale across the study population. As illustrated in Figure 3, significant declines were observed for three of the four relationship quality indicators (communication, interpersonal treatment, and patient trust). One aspect of relationship quality increased significantly (doctor's knowledge of the patient). Two of four organizational features of care showed significant change – one improvement (visit-based continuity, 1.2 points) and one decline (organizational access, −2.7 points). The other two organizational features of care were unchanged over the three years.

Figure 3
Changes in Doctor Patient Relationship Quality, 1996–1999

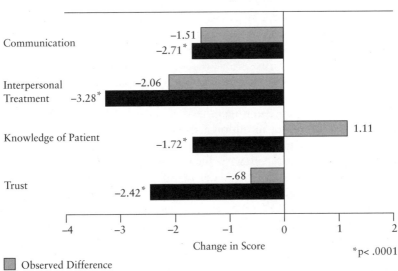

The decline in three of four relationship quality elements was unexpected and contrary to previous findings, which suggest that clinician-patient relationships that endure show gradual and continuous improvement. In fact, analyses that took into account the additional three years of the primary care relationship (1996–1999) suggested that all four relationship quality elements had "effective declines" that were substantially larger than the raw change scores reported above. That is, when analyses accounted for the primary care relationship duration, all four indicators of relationship quality were significantly lower in 1999 than had been expected based on the three additional years of doctor-patient interaction in each dyad.

It is unclear whether the observed decline in relationship quality is part of a trend that was occurring before we entered the field (1996) and/or whether it has continued since we exited (1999). However, the magnitude of the observed declines in this three-year period is equivalent to the erosion of approximately 10 per cent of the observed range of scores. This suggests the importance of continuing to measure and monitor the trajectory of physician-patient relationship quality in a health care delivery environment that continues to evolve and change.

Accounting for the observed changes in doctor-patient relationship quality. We generated eight hypotheses that might account for the observed decline in relationship quality. The study data (including those obtained from physicians in 1997 under the AHCPR-funded phase of the study) afford information to address seven of these hypotheses. We have completed those analyses and are now refining the information and preparing a manuscript in which to report the findings. Table 7 summarizes the hypotheses and what we found concerning each.

In summary, of the eight hypothesized drivers of relationship quality changes, we had data to address seven. Of these seven, three appear to have played a significant role. These were: (1) changes in the amount of time that patients had with their primary physician during office visits, (2) changes in visit-based continuity, and (3) changes in patients' disease burden. The changes in visit-based continuity appear to have countered the effects of time and disease burden. That is, visit-based continuity increased, on average, for patients in this study – and the observed increases in visit-based continuity appear to have helped to forestall larger declines in relationship quality that would have been observed in the absence of these continuity increases. The other two factors (time and disease burden), both appear to have contributed to the observed decline in relationship quality between 1996 and 1999.

Table 7
Explaining the observed decline in relationship quality: A summary of analyses

Hypothesized influence on relationship quality (RQ)	Hypothesized direction of effect on RQ	Analytic approach	Findings	Magnitude of effect
(1) Changes in *amount of time* MD spends with patient in visits	Negative	Patients' assessments of adequacy of time MD spends and of changes in time spent 1996–99 modelled as predictors of change in relationship quality scales	There was compelling evidence that changes in the amount of time spent with patients (perceived and reported by patients) was a significant driver of the reduced RQ observed in 1999 vs. 1996.	Changes in time accounted for an approximately 0.2– 0.25 point decline in RQ scales (largest of all observed effects).
(2) *Turmoil* in certain health plans	Negative	Comparison of changes in RQ reported by patients in plans that experienced extreme turmoil during the study period *vs.* those that did not	There was no evidence that plan turmoil had an effect on the observed changes in relationship quality. Patients in plans with and without turmoil showed equivalent change in all four elements of RQ.	None
(3) Changes in *patients' expectations*	Negative	Analysis of report-rating item pairs to see if patient expectations changed (e.g., was there lower rating of a given experience – for example, ten-minute office wait – in 1999 vs. 1996).	There was minimal evidence that patients' expectations concerning their care changed during the study period.	Minimal to none

Table 7
Explaining the observed decline in relationship quality: A summary of analyses (Continued)

Hypothesized influence on relationship quality (RQ)	Hypothesized direction of effect on RQ	Analytic approach	Findings	Magnitude of effect
(4) Changes in expectations of a subgroup of patients (higher socio-economic status, SES)	Negative	Analysis of high-SES subgroup vs. other patients to determine if that group is more demanding and if the pattern changed over the study period	There is evidence that the high-SES group is more demanding regarding their care, but this effect appeared to remain constant over the study period and therefore does not explain the observed decline in RQ.	None
(5) Decline in physician morale	Negative	Analysis of satisfaction data from the primary physicians whose patients participated in the study to see if an MD's satisfaction predicts his/her patients' assessments of care and/or predicts changes in patients' assessments of care	Physician satisfaction did not significantly predict his/her patients' assessments of care. There was no effect cross-sectionally or longitudinally. While we observed substantial declines in physician satisfaction (Murray et al. 2000a), physicians appear to have buffered their patients from their increasing dissatisfaction with their professional lives.	None
(6) Increase in visit-based continuity	Positive	Analysis of changes in visit-based continuity as predictors of changes in RQ scales	Changes in visit-based continuity significantly predicted changes in all four measures of RQ.	Changes in continuity corresponded with 0.14–0.22 point increases in RQ scales (i.e., the increased continuity experienced in many settings offset the other factors that were driving RQ downward).

Table 7
Explaining the observed decline in relationship quality: A summary of analyses (Continued)

Hypothesized influence on relationship quality (RQ)	Hypothesized direction of effect on RQ	Analytic approach	Findings	Magnitude of effect
(7) Occurrence of salient health event, acquisition of new medical conditions	Negative	Analysis of changes in the number and types of chronic medical conditions that patients reported over the study period as predictors of change in their assessments of their physicians' performance	Acquisition of new health conditions was associated with significant declines in patients' assessments of their physician – particularly in the relationship quality elements and integration of care.	Increased disease burden accounted for an approximately 0.1 point decline in RQ scales.
(8) Patients' feeling "stuck" – feeling a lack of options	Negative	No data to allow explicit study of this hypothesis	Our population had increasing choice available to them over the study course, so if they felt stuck, it was due to concerns about "the devil you know vs. the devil you don't" rather than due to the imposition of constraints on their choice of MD.	Unknown

Source: Copyright 2001 Tufts-New England Medical Center. Reprinted, with permission of the publisher, from D.G. Safran, Primary Care Performance: Views from the Patient: A Background Paper Prepared for the Robert Wood Foundation Meeting on the Future of Primary Care (Boston, MA: Tufts-New England Medical Center, 2001), 17–18.

SUMMARY

Demand for information about health care quality, and for tools with which to measure quality, has increased sharply in the past decade. The demand is fueled partly by public and private sector purchasers of health insurance, including employers, who want to assure the value being received for their expenditures. It is also fueled by a public that increasingly desires information with which to make good health care choices, particularly in the face of the continuing drive for cost containment that causes many to worry about whether their providers will have the incentives and ability to give them the best available care. Finally, it is fueled by health care organizations and clinicians that, in seeking to improve the quality of the care that they provide, recognize the need to measure and monitor performance with respect to many dimensions of care.

In this context, the Primary Care Assessment Survey (PCAS) is a valuable tool capable of providing patients, clinicians, health care organizations, purchasers, and policy makers with information about several important elements of quality. The Primary Care Assessment Survey is a brief, patient-completed questionnaire that measures each of seven defining features of primary care. The PCAS advances substantially beyond previous patient-based assessment tools, including our own (Safran et al. 1994b), by measuring features of care not previously assessed, including the physician's contextual (whole-person) knowledge of the patient, the patient's trust in the physician, and the physician's integration (coordination and synthesis) of the patient's care. Extensive psychometric testing of the instrument and scales demonstrate their strong psychometric performance in a general adult population and in sixteen population subgroups defined according to age, sex, race, years of education, household income, and health status (Safran et al. 1998d).

This chapter summarizes findings from one longitudinal study that used the PCAS to measure the quality of primary care in a general population of insured, employed adults, to identify characteristics of organizations and individuals that are associated with performance differences, and to examine the relationship between primary care performance and important outcomes of care. The study found that primary care performance differed significantly across five models of managed care (plan types) in ways that are consistent with and add to previous research on this issue. Overall, performance was most favourable in open-model delivery systems (i.e., those that do not contract with physicians on an exclusive basis) (Ware 1978a; Ware and Davies 1983). Staff-model HMOs performed least favourably on most measures. Among measured characteristics of patients, physicians, and health plans, health plan type was the variable associated with the largest observed differences in primary care performance.

Measured characteristics of physicians (age, sex, medical specialty, work load) were only modestly related to primary care performance. However, variance components methods revealed that these "fixed effects" models can be misleading. In variance components models, physicians accounted for a large portion of the variance in primary care performance measures – even though the specific physician characteristics that account for this remain elusive (Safran et al. 1998a; Safran et al. 1999). Future research is needed to identify characteristics of physicians that were not captured by discrete, measured variables in this study but that account for these substantial effects.

Future research must also seek to better understand the substantial relationship that was observed between patients' immediate social environments (as indicated by their census block groups) and the quality of primary care received (Safran et al. 1998a; Safran et al. 1999). And we must continue to explore the basis for the large interaction effects observed between patients' sociodemographic profiles and the identifiers denoting their primary physicians, sites of care, and health plans (Safran et al. 1999). Both of these findings suggest that the primary care received and reported by patients is substantially influenced by characteristics of the patients themselves. While these findings arose through the application of new analytic methods in this study, the methods are easily incorporated and applied in other health services research studies. As the field struggles to understand and address inequalities in health across our population, and to understand the role played by inequalities in health *care*, the potential value of routinely incorporating methods such as these into our research is clear.

Finally, the substantial relationship between primary care performance and outcomes of care that was observed in this study is important (Safran et al. 1998b). We continue to examine the relationship between primary care performance, as measured by the PCAS, and important outcomes of care (Barr 1995; AMA Council on Ethical and Judicial Affairs 1995). With the establishment of specific linkages between primary care performance and outcomes, the value of the information provided by the PCAS will be amplified. Not only will the instrument afford patients, clinicians, health care organizations, purchasers, and policy makers a detailed performance profile on essential and defining features of primary care, but it will also serve as a prognostic indicator of the outcomes that can be anticipated in the context of a particular level of primary care performance. That is, through results of longitudinal studies now underway, one can expect that it will ultimately be possible for clinicians, practice groups, and health plans to project any of several important outcomes of care based on their current PCAS performance profiles. In addition, by identifying those specific features of primary care, from among many, that are most predictive of outcomes, this work will guide priority setting for quality improvement initiatives. As these linkages between primary care performance and outcomes are elucidated, it is possible that the measurement and monitoring of primary care performance will prove to be one of the most versatile and informative tools available to the quality assessment field.

3

The Emotional and Interpersonal Dimensions of Health Care and Their Impact on Organizational and Clinical Outcomes: Building an Integrative, Action-Oriented Research Agenda[1]

CAROLE A. ESTABROOKS

INTERNATIONAL STUDY OF HOSPITAL ORGANIZATION AND NURSE OUTCOMES

This chapter centres around an international study of hospital organization and nurse outcomes presently being conducted in five countries, including Canada. The purpose of this study is to determine the impact of hospital organization and staffing on patient and nurse outcomes. The international study was launched in response to widespread hospital restructuring and work redesign, as well as to changing hospital staffing patterns – all of which were undertaken without empirical evidence of their effects on patient and system outcomes. The five participating countries are Canada (represented by British Columbia, Ontario, and Alberta), the United States (represented by Pennsylvania), England, Scotland, and Germany. The lead investigator is Dr Linda Aiken, a nurse and sociologist from the University of Pennsylvania. This chapter begins with an overview of the Canadian context of the study – and, more specifically, the Albertan context for health restructuring – and concludes with a discussion of early results from the Alberta study. The author would like to acknowledge the financial support provided by the Alberta Heritage Foundation for Medical Research, which made the Alberta portion of this international project possible.

---

1 The author would like to acknowledge the significant contribution of Kathryn Hesketh, MSc, in revising this paper.

THE CANADIAN CONTEXT

Among other things, Canada is known for "socialized medicine," commonly referred to as Medicare. While it is somewhat misleading to think of the Canadian health system as purely socialized, it is nonetheless true that this system differs significantly from American and other health care systems. The modern form of the Canadian system arose from the 1957 Hospital Insurance and Diagnostic Services Act, which was intended to ensure that no Canadian would lose home or financial security as a result of sickness. In 1984, the Canada Health Act was adopted, followed in 1996 by the Canada Health and Social Transfer Act (a block transfer of funds for health and social programs). In Canada, although health is a provincial jurisdiction, the federal government contributes a significant, albeit declining, proportion of provincial health dollars in the form of transfer payments. Those transfer payments constitute the primary lever by which the federal government enforces the Canada Health Act.

Any discussion of Medicare or the Canada Health Act must be founded on the five pillars of the system: universality, comprehensiveness, accessibility, portability, and public administration. However, the extent to which these principles are embedded in the Canadian psyche and function emblematically is not often explained. Recently, John Ralston Saul described Medicare as a metaphor for being Canadian (Saul 1998). He argues that while Canadians have difficulty describing what makes them fundamentally distinct from other nations, Medicare, and the principles and values that underpin it, capture and symbolize much of what it means to be Canadian. This identification with Medicare would, in part, explain the often visceral reaction to the extensive, and what some would describe as extreme, approach to health care restructuring (and to Bill 11) that occurred in Alberta in the mid nineties. This restructuring has repeatedly been accompanied by public/private funding tensions – with thinly disguised governmental interest (at least in Alberta) in increasing the proportion of private and third-party health care funding (Grant and Tiessen 1995).

Towards the end of 1992, with the election of Ralph Klein as leader of the Alberta Progressive Conservatives, Albertans became aware that a serious change was on the horizon. When the changes to health care came, they were swift, deep, and harsh (Cairney 1997; Gilmour 1994a; Maurier and Northcott 2000). In a very short period of time (with 1994 being the eye of the storm), the provincial health care system devolved from over 200 hospital boards to seventeen Regional Health Authorities and seventeen Regional Health Authority Boards (Alberta Health 1994; Maurier and Northcott 2000; Sutcliffe, Deber, and Pasut 1997). In addition, there were significant bed closures and thousands of nurse layoffs (Marck 1996). Health care providers endured a period of intense cuts in which a major ideological shift occurred under the guise of fiscal restraint (Lisac 1994; Wilson 2000). It is in this context that the Alberta research team joined an international team of investigators on the Study of Hospital Outcomes.

MODEL FOR THE INTERNATIONAL STUDY

The model for the study is presented in Table 1. The study comprises a series of independent replications rather than a large-scale pooling of the data, followed by a series of analyses. The data sources include: (1) primary data collected in a census of nurses, the variables being demographics, work environment, and nurse outcomes such as burnout, nurse abuse, job/career satisfaction, quality measures, and violence (note: this paper focuses on an analysis of this primary data); (2) secondary administrative data from sources such as the Canadian Institute for Health Information and Hospital Separation 1 and 2 Vital Statistics, including staffing records, patient mortality, failure to rescue, and length of stay. These data continue to be collected in several sites. Table 2 gives a sense of the magnitude of the sample.

Participating provinces have obtained their survey samples by various means. In Alberta a census was drawn of all staff nurses who identified on their annual registration (licensing) forms that they worked in a hospital. Four mailings were done using Dillman's (1991) methods between September 1998 and February 1999, resulting in a 53 per cent return rate.

The survey's 197 questions were the same for the seven study sites, with the exception of the final section, which contained province or site-specific questions. The survey sections were: (1) employment characteristics; (2) Nursing Work Index, revised (NWI-R); (3) the Maslach Burnout Inventory (MBI) characteristics; (4) characteristics of last shift; (5) demographics; (6) site-specific questions.

EXPLORATION OF THREE
OUTCOME VARIABLES

The analysis included in this chapter represents an exploration of three selected outcome variables – job and career satisfaction, workplace violence, and burnout (as per the Maslach Burnout Inventory; Maslach, Jackson, and Leiter 1996). To see if there were differences between major categories of nursing specialties (i.e., medical/surgical, critical care, and emergency) nurses were compared based on selected variables. Data at the individual level, rather than at the aggregated hospital level, were explored. Future analyses will include description and modelling at the aggregated hospital level.

Table 1
Model of the international study on the effect of hospital organization
on nurse and patient outcomes

Organizational structure and practice environment	→	Nurse outcomes	→	Patient outcomes
Examples:		Examples:		Examples:
Team relationships		Burnout		Mortality
Staffing resources		Job satisfaction		Failure to rescue
Nurse control over practice		Needle sticks		Length of stay

Table 2
International study sample

	Hospitals	Nurses
Canada – Alberta	109	6,526
Canada – British Columbia	97	2,838
Canada – Ontario	209	8,229
England	32	5,006
Germany	30	4,000
Scotland	27	5,238
USA – Pennsylvania	210	14,145
Total	714	46,531

Job and Career Satisfaction

Generally speaking, nurses in the survey are quite satisfied with their jobs, which is somewhat surprising. However, there are differences between the specialty areas: the percentage of nurses "satisfied and very satisfied with their present job" ranges from 77 per cent for those working in critical care areas, to 70 per cent for those in medical/surgical, to 67 per cent for those in emergency departments.

Comparison of the patterns for job satisfaction to career satisfaction (i.e., satisfaction with being a nurse) indicates that nurses are very satisfied with their career choices, despite the upheaval in the mid-1990s. (There were relatively small differences between nursing specialty groups.) However, nurses are also significantly less satisfied with their current jobs than they are with their overall career choice. There is a particularly large difference between job and career satisfaction for nurses in the medical/surgical areas. Table 3 shows that when only those nurses who said they were "very satisfied" are included, there are greater differences than when the "satisfied" and "very satisfied" categories are combined

Table 3
Job and career satisfaction

By specialty	Job satisfaction (% very satisfied)	Career satisfaction (% very satisfied)	Job satisfaction (% satisfied and very satisfied)	Career satisfaction (% satisfied and very satisfied)
Total	22	39	72	80
Med./Surg.	18	40	70	71
Critical care	26	37	77	79
Emergency	24	41	67	79

Source: Alberta Registered Nurse Survey, 1998 (n = 6,526).

When examining the results, it is important to remember that the nurses in this survey are survivors of the deep cuts of the nineties. In the mid-1990s many nurses were lost – some to the United States, some to other jobs, and some to early retirement (Loyie 1994). Between 1993 and 1995, it is estimated that between 2,000 and 3,000 nursing jobs were cut in Alberta, a loss of 15–20 per cent of the nursing workforce, with the bulk of the cuts being newly graduated (and by inference, the youngest) nurses (Gilmour 1994b). As of 1998, 43 per cent of Alberta RNs were forty-five years of age or older. By comparison, in 1993, only 35.7 per cent were in that age range (Alberta Association of Registered Nurses 2001). The impact on the health system of losing a large cadre of young nurses has not yet been measured; however, in light of the increasingly intense demographic pressures exerted by the baby boomers, and in light of nurses' earlier retirement choices, it seems clear that the loss will be significant (Ryten 1997).

Workplace Violence

In the survey, a section was reserved for site-specific questions. In Alberta, a series of questions related to workplace violence was included. Violence against nurses was defined in several ways, as presented in Table 4. Specific definitions and examples were given prior to asking the nurses to select a response for each kind of violence. To get a sense of the acuity of the problem, as well as to ensure accuracy of reporting, nurses were asked to answer based on the *past five shifts that they had worked.*

In subsequent questions, nurses were asked to specify the source of the abuse and whether they had reported the episode. Additional questions asked nurses: (1) the extent to which they agreed with the statement that their employer had taken measures to address violence in the workplace; (2) to evaluate how their emotional well-being fared

Table 4
Abuse and assault of nurses

Type of assault	Examples
Physical assault	Being spit on, bitten, hit, pushed
Threat of assault	Verbal or written threats intending harm
Emotional abuse	Insults, gestures, humiliation before the work team, coercion
Verbal sexual harassment	Repeated, unwanted, intimate questions or remarks of a sexual nature
Sexual assault	Any forced physical/sexual contact, including forcible touching and fondling, or any forced sexual act, including forcible intercourse

compared to one year ago; and (3) to indicate how often they feared for their personal safety while carrying out their responsibilities as a registered nurse.

Many nurses experienced abuse. The main findings are the frequencies with which Alberta nurses reported experiencing one or more types of abuse. These are presented in Table 5 below. An alarming 46 per cent of nurses in the sample had experienced one or more types of violence in the past five shifts they had worked. The frequency of experienced violence varies from one form of violence to another. There were also significant differences among the seventeen regions in Alberta, with some regions having almost no violence and others having high rates of violent episodes. While regional variation is somewhat disconcerting, it is also an indication that factors like policy implementation at the regional level have an impact on violence against nurses.

Emotional abuse is the most common form of workplace violence with a rate of 381 per 1,000 Alberta nurses per five shifts worked. It is followed by threats of assault at 177 per 1,000 nurses, physical assaults at 169 per 1,000 nurses, verbal sexual abuse at seventy-seven per 1,000 nurses, and sexual assault at a rate of five per 1,000 Alberta nurses.

Patients were the most frequent "perpetrators." When asked who had been the source of the violence, nurses very frequently cited patients as the abusers. They were the source of 98% of physical assaults, 83% of threats of physical assault, 81% of sexual assaults, and 67% of verbal sexual harassment. The sources of emotional abuse were more evenly distributed, with 35% being attributed to patients, 13% to physicians, 13% to nursing co-workers, 12% to patient families and visitors, 10% to a combination of patient and family, and 14% to multiple sources.

Table 5
Alberta nurses who experienced abuse/assault in past five shifts

Type of violence experienced	Rate per 1,000 nurses
Emotional abuse	381
Threat of assault	177
Physical assault	169
Verbal sexual abuse	77
Sexual assault	5

Source: Alberta Registered Nurse Survey, 1998 (n = 6,526).

Nurses often did not report abuse. The nurses surveyed were asked if they had reported any of the violence they had experienced. Of those who had been a victim of one or more types of violence in the past five shifts worked, 67% did not report the incident. The level of reporting varied according to the type of violence; threats were most often reported (40% of cases), whereas only 29% of the emotional abuse and 24% of the verbal sexual harassment was reported. The level of reporting also varied between specialty areas. As an example, the reporting of emotional abuse was less frequent in medical/surgical, critical care, and emergency nursing (ranging from 22% to 29%) than in other units (with ranges from 31% to 35%). This survey did not address the issues surrounding why nurses fail to report abuse, but it is an important question that needs to be answered in order for hospital management to be able to adequately address violence in the workplace. For further reference to analyses on workplace violence in Alberta hospitals, please refer to Duncan et al. 2001 and Hesketh et al. forthcoming.

Burnout

Another nursing outcome examined was burnout, as measured by the Maslach Burnout Inventory (MBI) (Maslach et al. 1996). Maslach and others have reported that burnout can lead to deterioration in the quality of care provided. It appears to be a factor in turnover, absenteeism, and low morale (Felton 1998). It also seems to be correlated with numerous self-reported indices of personal dysfunction, including insomnia, headaches, and stress-related illness (Cole 1992).

Maslach's Burnout Inventory includes three subscales: personal achievement, emotional exhaustion, and depersonalization.The inventory evaluates each individual's experience, on a continuum from burnout to engagement with work, by means of the distinct assessment of three components: (1) the impact on emotional and creative energy;

(2) the impact on personal accomplishment; and (3) the degree of depersonalization and cynicism about work. Overall, on the total burn-out score, which is a sum of the three subscales, differences between specialty groups were significant, as shown in Table 6. Emergency nurses reported the highest overall scores. Perhaps of greater interest is how much lower critical care nurses are on the scale, compared to those in emergency or medical/surgical, particularly on the emotional exhaustion and depersonalization scores. The Burnout Inventory behaved very much as Maslach suggests it should, with relatively low correlation between personal accomplishment and the other two scales, and a relatively high correlation between depersonalization and emotional exhaustion. In this sample, each of the subscales had high alpha coefficients: 0.9 for the items on the emotional exhaustion subscale and 0.8 for the other two

Analysis of variables that predict emotional exhaustion. As a final set of preliminary analyses, a simple regression analysis model using selected variables that predict a nurse's emotional exhaustion was created. Consistent with Maslach's recommendation that subscales be treated separately, and given that "emotional exhaustion" had performed well in earlier work conducted by Aiken and others (Aiken and Sloane 1997; Aiken, Sloane, and Sochalski 1998), this factor was chosen as the outcome variable. Eight variables were selected that we thought would contribute to emotional exhaustion. The eight variables were: hours worked, number of shift changes during the past two weeks, management resolving reported problems, good working relationships with physicians, not having to do things against one's nursing judgment, enough staff to get the work done, magnitude of overtime increases, and specialty area.

A simple regression model accounted for 30 per cent of the variance in emotional exhaustion. Only predictors related to the immediate work context were selected for this model. Clearly, however, emotional exhaustion is influenced by multiple factors, many of which are beyond the work context. Given that questions on the emotional exhaustion subscale are not all restricted to the work context, and given the complex nature of emotional exhaustion, creating a model that accounts for almost one-third of the variation in this variable is important for its explanatory potential.

Typical cases. A comparison of the emotional exhaustion a nurse experiences with varying environmental factors illustrates the utility of this model to hospital decision makers. For example, in both case 1 and case 2 (see Table 7), the typical nurse works on a medical/surgical unit for an average of thirty hours per week. Almost everything in the

Table 6
Alberta registered nurses mean scores, Maslach Burnout Inventory (MBI)

Specialty area	Personal accomplishment (failure to have sense of)	Emotional exhaustion	Depersonalization	Total
Emergency	10	24	11	45
Med./surg.	11	23	7	41
Multiple units	11	22	7	50
Critical care	10	20	5	35
All other units	10	21	5	36
Psychiatry	9	19	5	33

Source: Alberta Registered Nurse Survey, 1998 (n = 6,526).

Table 7
Organizational features and emotional exhaustion

Med./surg. nurse (case 1)	Med./surg. nurse (case 2)
–7.25 constant	–7.25 constant
+ 0.17 × 30-hour week (30)	+ 0.17 × 30-hour week (30)
+ 3.57 × strongly disagree there is enough staff (4)	+ 3.57 × strongly agrees there is enough staff (1)
+ 1.91 × medical surgical (1)	+ 1.91 × medical surgical (1)
+ 0 × not critical care (0)	+ 0 × not critical care (0)
+ 1.61 × emergency (0)	+ 1.61 × emergency (0)
+ 0.26 × 1 shift changes in the past two weeks (1)	+ 0.26 × shift changes in the past two weeks (1)
+ 1.58 × somewhat agrees good Dr-RN working relationship (2)	+ 1.58 × Somewhat agrees good Dr-RN working relationship (2)
+ 1.72 × very confident mgmt will resolve pt. problems (1)	+ 1.72 × very confident mgmt will resolve pt. problems (1)
+ 2.07 × somewhat agrees not asked to do things against nurse's judgment (2)	+ 2.07 × somewhat agrees not asked to do things against nurse's judgment (2)
+ 1.64 × overtime decreased from previous year (–1)	+ 1.64 × overtime decreased from previous year (–1)
Emotional exhaustion = 21.8	Emotional exhaustion = 12.7

nurse's unit reflects a reasonably constructive, positive practice environment. The only difference between the two cases is that, in case 1, there is "inadequate staff to do the work," whereas in case 2 there is "adequate staff to do the work."

In case 1 (inadequate staffing), the nurse finds herself at the end of any given day in the mid-range of exhaustion (at 21.8) that she and her peers will experience. While it is not known what set of behavioural consequences are associated with any given score or range of scores, it is likely that continuous emotional exhaustion in the mid-range would result in some degree of cumulative and detrimental effect on the quality of nursing care delivered.

In case 2 (adequate staffing), the nurse's emotional exhaustion level drops to a level well into the lower third of scores (at 12.7). The importance of having "enough staff to do the job" is crucial, as any practising nurse on any unit will indicate. However, it is reasonable to expect that resource adequacy and other workplace elements will persist as important influences on patient outcomes as analysis progresses.

CONCLUSION

A relatively simple model, such as the one presented above, is limited in that it does not capture the complexities of the practice environment. The aim of the Hospital Outcomes Study is to eventually use more complex modelling techniques to explore the relationships between the practice environment, including an organization's structural characteristics, and nurse, patient, and ultimately system outcomes. However, as illustrated in Table 1, nurse outcomes represent a "black box" by which an organization influences such patient outcomes as mortality and "failure to rescue" (Silber and Rosenbaum 1997). Even this relatively simple model suggests the importance of selecting practice environment characteristics that directly influence the working nurse. It also hints at the potential of this work to demonstrate the impact of organizational factors and the practice environment on nurse outcomes. These outcomes are frequently *emotional or psychological* in nature and consequently are often undervalued as powerful predictors of patient outcomes.

As more analyses emerge from this international study of nurse and hospital outcomes, it becomes clear that the well-being of nurses is highly dependent on the quality of their hospital work environment (Duncan et al. 2001; Estabrooks et al. 2002; Hesketh et al. 2001), including factors like support, adequacy of resources, and interpersonal relationships. Furthermore, analyses linking nursing to patient outcomes suggest that when nursing work conditions are poor, not only are nurses at risk, but so are patients (Aiken, Clarke, Sloane, Sochalski, and Silber 2002; Needleman, Buerhaus, Mattke, Stewart, and Zelevinsky 2002).

Given the current predictions of massive nurse shortages in Alberta and the rest of Canada (Canadian Nurses Association 1997), it is critical that these issues be addressed by institutions and policy makers. Failure to do so will adversely affect our ability to retain a vital and healthy nursing workforce.

4

Measuring and Monitoring
Patient Outcomes

DIANE M. IRVINE DORAN

The measurement of outcomes has gained in importance as health care organizations focus on the areas of cost and quality, effectiveness of care, and organizational performance. All practitioners in the health field are being challenged to find ways to demonstrate that the care they provide leads to improved outcomes for the recipients of that care. To do so, health care practitioners are attempting to identify relevant outcomes that can be linked in a meaningful way to their practices.

Nursing, like the other health disciplines, has responded to this challenge through a number of initiatives, such as the American Nurses' Association Report Card (1997), the Nursing Component of the Ontario Hospital Report Card (McGillis Hall, Irvine Doran, Laschinger, Mallette, and O'Brien-Pallas 2001a), and empirical research demonstrating a relationship between nursing care and patient outcomes (Irvine Doran, O'Brien-Pallas, Sidani, McGillis Hall, Petryshen, and Watt-Watson 2001; McGillis Hall, Irvine Doran, Baker, Pink, Sidani, O'Brien-Pallas, and Donner 2001b).

In this chapter, I review some of the key findings from the literature on outcomes assessment in health care and focus specifically on the literature that has examined the impact of the emotional and interpersonal dimensions of health care on patient outcome achievement. A conceptual model is proposed to explain how the emotional dimensions of work can impact on the quality of patient care and outcome achievement. Finally, the results of a study that examined the influence of nursing staff job satisfaction on patient outcomes in an acute care setting is presented. Although the material for the chapter draws on examples from the nursing literature, the concepts presented and issues raised are relevant for understanding the relationship between the emotional dimensions of work and patient outcomes for all health care disciplines.

THE RELATIONSHIP BETWEEN NURSE JOB SATISFACTION AND PATIENT OUTCOMES

The affective response of health care providers to their work environment and its impact on their interactions with other providers and patients has become a topic of interest because of the increased focus on the cost and quality of health care. Job satisfaction is a component of the provider's affective response to the work environment (Irvine Doran and Evans 1995). A relationship between the job satisfaction of providers and the outcomes for patients has been empirically demonstrated on numerous occasions. In 1981, Holland, Konick, and Buffum found that in hospitals where staff participation was high, practitioners reported higher levels of job satisfaction. This, in turn, was associated with better post-hospital adjustment by patients than was exhibited by those discharged from hospitals where participation and satisfaction levels were low. In a study involving seventy-seven family planning clinics, Weisman and Nathanson (1985) found that the job satisfaction level of nursing staff was the strongest predictor of the satisfaction level of clients, which in turn was the strongest predictor of the rate of clients' contraceptive compliance. Linn, Brook, Clark, Davies, Fink, and Kosecoff (1985) found a similar relationship between the satisfaction levels of physicians and clients and that the increased satisfaction of both had economic, psychological, and social benefits. Mitchell, Armstrong, Simpson, and Lentz (1989) found that the job satisfaction of nurses working in intensive care units affected the quality of patient care. Furthermore, higher quality care was associated with fewer complications experienced by patients and with higher patient satisfaction. More recently, a Canadian study conducted by Leiter, Harview, and Frizzell (1998) revealed that patients were more satisfied when nurses found their work meaningful. Patients were less satisfied when nursing staff felt more exhausted or when nurses expressed an intention to leave their work place.

Although these studies varied in research design, setting, and outcomes examined, they each offer evidence that a relationship exists between the health provider's affective response to the work situation, the quality of care provided, and the outcomes of care for patients. Weisman and Nathanson (1985) suggested an explanation for the relationship between provider job satisfaction and the quality of care. They noted that the nature of health care work, which involves high levels of direct client contact, is dependent on the interpersonal quality of the provider-client interaction. "[A] health professional who is more satisfied with his or her working conditions may interact more effectively with clients because the positive affect associated with high job satisfaction has a spillover effect on the provider's interactions with clients. Conversely, providers who are dissatisfied with their working conditions might find it difficult to put aside their own problems to deal effectively with those of the client" (Weisman and Nathanson 1985, 1,180). This causal chain is depicted below in the top row of Figure 1.

Another plausible explanation for the relationship observed between staff job satisfaction and client outcomes is depicted in the bottom row of Figure 1. Staff dissatisfaction with their jobs can lead to increased staff absenteeism and staff turnover (Irvine Doran and Evans 1995). This, in turn, can lead to fragmented staffing because of the need to replace full-time staff with casual staff. Fragmented staffing disrupts the continuity of care and, along with reliance on reduced or less experienced staff, can increase the probability that a patient will experience an adverse occurrence resulting in secondary complications associated with the hospital stay. For instance, Williams and Murphy (1979) found that the adequacy of staffing affected the quality of nurse communication with the patient and/or family and the thoroughness of the nurse's observation of the patient. Behner, Fogg, Fournier, Frankenbach, and Robertson (1990) found that staffing at 20 per cent below the recommended level during the first three days of a patient's stay resulted in a 30 per cent increase in the probability that the patient would experience a complication while in the hospital, which in turn would lead to an additional 3.5 days of hospital stay

Figure 1
Causal mechanisms linking job satisfaction and outcomes

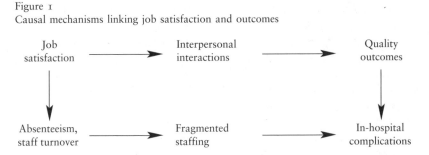

Thus job satisfaction impacts on interpersonal interactions that, in turn, affect outcomes. Low job satisfaction also results in absenteeism and staff turnover, which can lead to fragmented staffing, an increased probability of in-hospital complications, and poor outcomes for patients.

ONTARIO STUDY

A study completed by Sidani and Irvine Doran (1999a) is useful for illustrating the relationship between nurse job satisfaction and patient outcomes in an acute care setting. The incentive for the study came from hospital restructuring and its impact both on the distribution of nurses within the acute care system (McGillis Hall 1997) and on the nature of nurses' work (Davidson, Folcarelli, Crawford, Dupart, and Clifford 1997). In particular, "hospital-based nurses in the 1990's have had to confront the dual demands of caring for sicker patients with fewer resources and smaller staffs" (Davidson et al. 1997, 635). In the first empirical examination of the effect of health care reform on nurses' job satisfaction and voluntary turnover, Davidson et al. (1997) reported a significant reduction in nurses' job satisfaction following hospital restructuring.

Irvine Doran, Sidani, and McGillis Hall (1998) developed a conceptual model to guide the assessment of nurses' contributions to health care and patient outcome achievement. This model was used to guide the selection of variables to be included in a study of the impact of hospital restructuring on the job satisfaction of nurses, the quality of care, and patient outcomes in an acute care hospital in Ontario.

The Nursing Role Effectiveness Model (Irvine Doran et al. 1998), depicted in Figure 2, relates the achievement of specific patient outcomes to the independent, dependent, and interdependent roles and functions assumed by nurses. The nurse's independent role entails the functions for which only nurses are held accountable. They include the activities of patient assessment, decision-making, intervention, and follow-up that define much of the direct contact nurses have with patients. The nurse's dependent role entails the activities and judgments associated with the implementation of medical orders and medical treatments. The nurse's interdependent role entails the activities and interactions in which nurses engage that promote the coordination and integration of the care provided by different professional and paraprofessional staff (Irvine Doran et al. 1998). The conceptual model identified a set of structural variables that affect (1) the nurse's capacity to engage in effective role performance and (2) the relationship between the nursing process and patient outcomes. These variables include the nurse's educational preparation, experience level, and tenure within the organization (Irvine Doran et al. 1998). They also include practice

Figure 2
The Nursing Role Effectiveness Model

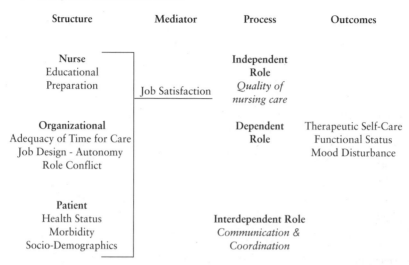

Structure	Mediator	Process	Outcomes

Source: Copyright 1998 Jannetti Publications Inc. Reprinted, with permission of the publisher, from D.M. Irvine Doran, S. Sidani, and L. McGillis Hall, "Linking outcomes to nurses' roles in health care," *Nursing Economic $* 16, no. 2 (1998): 59.

setting variables such as the staff mix, the care delivery model, job autonomy, and the clarity of role definition and responsibilities (Irvine Doran et al. 1998). Sidani and Irvine Doran (1999b) adapted the model to the evaluation of the acute care nurse's role.

The study we conducted expanded on the examination of the relationships proposed in the Nursing Role Effectiveness Model by evaluating the mediating role of nurses' job satisfaction. The central idea tested in this study was that the effect of the unit structural variables on nurses' role performance is mediated by nurses' job satisfaction. A mediator variable represents the generative mechanism through which independent variables influence the dependent variable of interest (Baron and Kenny 1986). Mediator variables help us to understand how or why such variables as job design affect outcomes such as nurses' role performance.

Design

A cross-sectional design was used to collect data on the unit structure, nursing process, and job satisfaction variables. The study received ethical approval from the hospital's Human Subjects Review Board. Data were collected through structured questionnaires. Table 1 provides

Table 1
Study instruments and data analysis study instruments

Instruments	
Structural variables	• Nurse and patient demographics • Job autonomy – Hackman and Oldham JDS (1980) (alpha 0.71) • Perceived role tension – Lyons (1971) (alpha 0.78) • Adequacy of time for care (alpha 0.89)
Process variables	• Nurses' independent role: Patient judgment of nursing care quality (alpha 0.94) • Nurses' interdependent role: Unit communications – Shortell et al. (1994) (alpha 0.85); and unit coordination – Shortell et al. (1994) (alpha 0.77)
Nurse outcome	• Job satisfaction (Job Descriptive Survey) (alpha 0.88)
Patient outcome	• Functional status (alpha 0.89) • Mood disturbance (alpha 0.82) • Therapeutic self-care (alpha 0.88)
Data analysis	• Structural equation modelling
Multiple levels of analysis	• Nurse and unit structural variables aggregated to the unit level • Patient structural and outcome variables measured at the individual level

information about the instruments used to collect data on the structural, process, and outcome variables, the approach to data analysis, and the unit of analysis.

Setting and Sample

The study was conducted in a large tertiary care treatment facility in southern Ontario consisting of 850 beds and located on two separate sites within the same metropolitan area. The sample consisted of nurses employed full-time and part-time on in-patient medical, surgical, and obstetrical units. Two hundred and fifty-four registered nurses (RNs) and registered practical nurses (RPNs) consented to participate and returned completed questionnaires. This represented approximately 35% of potential participants. Because participation was confidential, it was not possible to follow-up with non-responders. Most of the nurses had a diploma from a community college program (53.3%). They were primarily female (90%) with an average age of thirty-eight years and an average tenure within the hospital of eleven years. The majority of the nurses worked rotating shits (56%). Eighty-two per cent were RNS, 4.4% care leaders, 2.6% RPNS, 1.8% nurse managers, and 1.1% unit clerks or patient care assistants (PCAS). Four per cent comprised other nursing staff associated with the unit, such as clinical nurse specialists and nurse educators.

Three hundred and seventy-two patients consented to participate in the study, for a response rate of approximately 73%. This represented approximately 49% of the patients who would have been eligible to participate, the remainder having been missed because they were away from the room or busy with the physician/nurse, or because they had already been discharged when data collection began. The average age of the patients was fifty-four years, with an almost even split between males (45%) and females (55%). The majority of patients had a high-school education (33%), were Anglo Saxon (56%), and were married (64%), and this was their first hospitalization for their current medical concern (80%). The predominant medical case mix groups (CMGs) were major cardiac procedures and conditions such as heart failure/coronary artery bypass surgery (18%), major gynaecological and colorectal procedures (13.8%), angina and/or cardiac catheterization (11.2%), orthopaedic procedures (7.5%), and asthma and pneumonia (4.5%).

The patient outcomes that were examined in this study included: (1) therapeutic self-care, which represented the patient's ability to manage the presenting health problem and involved self-observation or monitoring, perception and recognition of symptoms or changes in functioning, and selection and performance of actions to relieve symptoms and to maintain or improve function; (2) the functional status of the patient, such as resuming daily activities following hospital discharge; and (3) mood disturbance, which included the patient's report of anger, sadness, anxiety, or confusion at the time of hospital discharge. Outcomes were risk adjusted for medical diagnosis and length of stay before assessing the effect of the nurse and unit structure variables, job satisfaction, and nurses' role performance on outcome achievement.

Study Results

The means, standard deviations, and zero-order correlation coefficients among the study variables are presented in Table 2. The standardized direct and total effects of each independent variable on the three dependent variables are presented in Table 3. The model had a good fit, as indicated by the values of the fit indices presented in Table 3.

The nurse and unit structure variables had significant direct effects on nurses' job satisfaction. Job autonomy had a positive effect on

Table 2
Means, standard deviations, and correlations among the study variables

	1 nurse education	2 patient age	3 job autonomy	4 role tension	5 time for care	6 job satisfaction	7 effectiveness of communications	8 effectiveness of nursing care	9 coordination of care	10 functional status	11 therapeutic self-care	12 mood disturbance
1												
2	-0.09	54.26 (17)										
3	-0.04	-0.01	5.09 (1.17)									
4	0.30***	-0.07	-0.32***	2.64 (0.66)								
5	-0.28***	0.08	-0.15**	-0.45***	1.80 (0.64)							
6	-0.10	0.10	0.74***	-0.57***	0.27***	4.55 (0.91)						
7	0.24***	0.05	0.31***	-0.36***	0.05	0.35***	3.48 (0.53)					
8	0.09	-0.02	0.11*	0.06	0.14**	-0.04	0.00	3.87 (0.65)				
9	0.16**	-0.07	0.09	-0.43***	0.19***	0.30***	0.51***	-0.14**	3.27 (0.56)			
10	0.05	-0.03	-0.003	0.01	-0.007	-0.03	0.04	0.19***	-0.03	2.75 (0.95)		
11	-0.008	-0.16**	0.05	-0.09	0.04	-0.005	0.11*	0.18***	-0.03	0.34***	4.36 (0.87)	
12	-0.03	-0.10	0.04	-0.08	0.03	0.03	-0.02	-0.19***	0.06	-0.09	-0.27***	1.68 (1.04)

*$p < 0.05$, **$p < 0.01$, ***$p < 0.001$

Table 3
The goodness of fit statistics for the relationships among the variables in the Nursing Role Effectiveness Model*

Dependent variables	Job satisfaction	Communication	Coordination	Quality of nurse care	Therapeutic self-care	Functional status	Mood disturbance
Standardized effects	Direct/Total	Direct/Total	Direct/Total	Direct/Total	Direct/Total	Direct/Total	Direct/Total
Patient age	0.06/0.06	–/0.01	-0.16/-0.14	–/0.02	-0.17/-0.16	–/-0.05	-0.15/-0.11
Nurse education	0.08/0.08	0.37/0.38	0.19/0.35	–/-0.06	–/-0.01	–/-0.01	–/-0.01
Job autonomy	0.72/0.72	–/0.12	-0.31/-0.08	–/0.01	–/0.03	–/0.01	–/-0.01
Role tension	-0.23/-0.23	-0.37/-0.41	-0.31/-0.52	–/0.09	-0.13/-0.09	–/-0.02	–/0.01
Time for care	0.30/0.30	–/-0.05	–/0.09	0.17/0.16	–/0.02	–/0.03	–/-0.03
Job satisfaction		0.17/0.17	0.25/0.32	–/-0.06	–/-0.03	–/-0.02	–/0.02
Communication			0.36/0.36	–/-0.06	0.15/0.08	–/-0.02	–/-0.02
Coordination				-0.18/-0.18	-0.15/-0.18	–/-0.08	–/0.07
Quality of nursing care					0.17/0.17	0.13/0.19	-0.14/-0.19
Therapeutic self-care						0.31/0.31	-0.27/-0.27

*Model

Model fit		
Chi-square	Root mean square residual	Adjusted goodness of fit
43.61 (p = 0.15, df 35)	0.15	0.96

nurses' job satisfaction, whereas role tension had a negative effect. The more highly the nurses were educated the more satisfied they were with their job. The adequacy of time to provide patient care was positively associated with nurses' job satisfaction. Nurses who cared on average for a greater number of older patients reported higher levels of job satisfaction than those who cared for mostly younger patients. Therefore, the hypothesized relationships between the nurse and unit structure variables and nurses' job satisfaction were supported.

The two work design variables, autonomy and role tension, also had a direct effect on nurses' interdependent role performance (i.e., on the effectiveness of nurse communications and coordination of care). The direction of the relationship suggests that communications are more effective when nurses have autonomy in their jobs and when their role responsibilities are clearly defined (i.e., when they do not experience role tension). In contrast, job autonomy had a negative effect on the coordination of care. Nurse education had a direct positive effect on the quality of nurse communications and the coordination of care. Nurses' job satisfaction mediated the effects of the adequacy of time for care and patient age on nurse communication. Nurses' job satisfaction had a positive effect on nurse communication and coordination of care. Therefore, the hypothesized effect of job satisfaction on nurses' interdependent role performance was supported. The two interdependent role variables, nurse communication and coordination of care, were interrelated. The perceived adequacy of time to provide care was the only structural variable to have a significant positive effect on nurses' independent role performance (measured as the patient's perception of the quality of nursing care).

The three role-performance variables had direct effects on one or more of the patient outcomes and, with the exception of patient age, fully mediated the effect of the nurse and unit structure variables on outcome achievement. These findings suggest that the unit structure variables and nurse job satisfaction affect the processes of care, which in turn affect the outcomes of care.

A closer look at the study results reveals that job satisfaction operates as a mediator variable for some, but not all, of the unit structure variables and that it affects the processes of care (i.e., role performance), which in turn affect the quality of the outcomes patients achieve at the time of hospital discharge.

DISCUSSION

Nurses' job satisfaction had a significant influence on the quality of nursing care, as reflected in the quality of nurses' communication with the other health care providers and in the coordination of care. These results underscore the importance of the emotional and interpersonal dimensions of health care. It behoves health care administrators not to neglect this important aspect of the providers' response to their environment when restructuring care services. The creation of working conditions that improve nurses' job satisfaction will have significant benefits not only in terms of the outcomes traditionally linked to job satisfaction, such as turnover and absenteeism (Irvine Doran and Evans 1995), but also in terms of the quality of nurses' role performance and the quality of patient outcomes.

The jobs health providers assume in hospitals need to be designed to promote autonomy and reduce role tension. In order to capitalize on their knowledge and skill level, staff need to be allowed discretion within their jobs to exercise independent judgment in patient care decisions and actions. Rigid job descriptions, close supervision, autocratic leadership, and formalized policies and procedures are organizational factors that have been identified as hindrances to worker autonomy and discretion (Conger and Kanungo 1988; Johns 1996).

The job satisfaction of providers is one aspect of their emotional response to the work situation. Their emotional response influences the quality of their interactions with others. Health care organizations are characterized by high levels of direct client contact, and the provider-client interaction is key to the performance of work in health care. The interpersonal quality of the provider-client interaction is important to the quality of care and to patient outcome achievement.

The results of this study support the causal relationship between job satisfaction and client outcomes suggested by Weisman and Nathanson (1985) and depicted in Figure 1. The results are consistent with two earlier studies conducted in the United States depicting the impact of team communications on patient outcomes. The first such study was conducted by Knaus, Draper, Wagner, and Zimmerman (1986) and was a prospective study of consecutive admissions of 5,030 patients to ICUs at thirteen tertiary care hospitals in the United States. Outcomes were risk adjusted using the Appache II risk classification system. Differences in expected death rates were related more to the interaction of each hospital's intensive care unit staff than to the amount of specialized treatment used or the hospital's teaching status. The second study, conducted by Shortell, Zimmerman, Rousseau, Gillies, Wagner, Draper, Knaus, and Duffy (1994), was a prospective follow-up of 17,440 patients across forty-two ICUs in the United States. Outcomes were risk adjusted using the Appache III risk classification system. Questionnaires assessing team relations, communication, and organizational performance were completed by 1,418 nurses and 790 physicians and residents. Caregiver interaction and communication were associated with a shorter risk-adjusted length of stay. These two studies, as well as the study described in this chapter, offer fairly compelling evidence that the quality of providers' interpersonal interactions is important to the quality of care and outcomes of care within health care organizations.

CONCLUSION

The results of this study confirm what was previously known about the relationship between staff job satisfaction and the quality of patient outcomes. The study expands our understanding of this relationship by explicating the way in which job satisfaction operates to influence patient outcomes. Specifically, job satisfaction partially mediates the effect of unit structure and staff variables on outcome variables and has a direct effect on the quality of work performance, which in turn affects patient outcomes. Hospital administrators run the risk of compromising the quality of patient care if they persist in hospital downsizing and restructuring without paying attention to the quality of the worklife of staff within their organizations.

5

Behind Every Great Caregiver: The Emotional Labour in Health Care

ARLIE RUSSELL HOCHSCHILD

Although I am a sociologist by training, my approach is an anthropological one. I interview and observe people over a fairly long period of time. It was on the basis of such a research approach that I introduced the term "emotional labour" to capture the emotional dimension of what is produced in most service industries (Hochschild 1979, 1983, 2003a; see Ashforth and Humphrey 1993 for a review of applications of the concept). While my early work focused on the emotional labour of airline employees, my current research is based on interviews with nannies, elderly care workers, and "ritual workers" – funeral parlour directors and wedding planners. I have also interviewed a half dozen doctors and nurses. Let me now explore what stands out from this diverse set of interviews about the emotional dimension of care.

DEFINING EMOTIONAL CARE

"Emotional care" is a generic term for a highly personal experience. Depending upon each caregiver and receiver, emotional care feels – and is – different. As my interviews suggest, those who give care, like those who receive it, are often at a loss to describe what they actually do when they "care." And little wonder; the culture itself provides us with a highly limited vocabulary with which to describe care. The words we have – care, like, help, feel responsible for – all beg the question: What exactly are we *doing, feeling,* and *thinking* while we're providing care, liking, helping, or feeling responsible?

Also, what is "care" from the recipient's point of view? One patient may experience care as "soothing." In what he or she says, in how slowly she moves, in the direction of her gaze, in every action, the nurse may reduce stimuli by focusing the patient's attention on something pleasing – in a word, "sooth." Another patient may experience care as empowerment. In how respectful she is of the patient's desire to know about an illness and in how mindful of the anxieties associated both with knowing and not knowing, a nurse may enhance the patient's sense of mastery. In a word, she may "empower." Yet another patient may experience care as encouragement. The nurse may remind, joke, or chastise the patient in such a way as to elicit hope. But whatever the *result* of a given interaction – relaxation, elation, encouragement – the nurse has expressed his or her care through *emotional attunement* to the patient's *needs*.

Attunement is a large part of emotional care, but it isn't all of it. As Joan Tronto argues in *Moral Boundaries*, we may "care about" (stay attuned), or "care for" (act on the basis of attunement), or do both simultaneously (Tronto 1993). A relative in Toledo, Ohio, may "care about" her dying mother, while a nurse in St Petersburg, Florida, may be caring for her. Here the distinction is between empathy and action, thought and practice.

A caretaker's attunement to the patient's needs – to focus on that for a moment – can vary in degree (is it more or less?), constancy (is it dependable or not?), and "projective load" (is it based on the needs of the patient or on some distorted perception of the patient?). By "projective load" I mean to say that every act of empathy ("I understand how you feel") comes with a projection ("I see you through the lens of my own experience"). That is, I see you *as like* something or someone I have experienced in the past. So a person might see "you" as "like my generous mother" or "like my depressed sister." With the act of empathy, then, comes the act of perception and projection. So, with any act of "our now" is a little bit of "my then." Clearly, some projections enhance care while others harm it. Indeed, psychiatrists – who receive specialized training in attunement – are taught to track and try to filter out the "my then" from the "our now" so as to more accurately hear what the patient him or herself really feels and needs.

In light of this, we can ask how the concept of emotional labour applies to emotional care by focusing on at least three things: (1) the degree of attunement (i.e., the effort we put into it); (2) the quality of attunement (i.e., the degree of accurate understanding of the other's experience); and (3) the reliability of attunement.

The caregiver is attuned to a need, oftentimes through a feeling. But we often learn about feelings through telling and listening to personal stories. As Christopher Wellin observes, the stories we tell each other are central to emotional communication (Wellin 2002).

The caregiver can attune himself to a story "from a distance." In this case, the story remains implicit, and references to it are curtailed or indirect. For example, one woman, a recovering alcoholic and a member of Alcoholics Anonymous (AA), described the support she received and gave through daily phone calls. In her words: "The person (whom she calls) will tell me a short story to which I will respond with a parallel story. No questions are asked; it's merely an exchange of stories which serve to make us all feel we are not alone in our situation." Such calls act as "boosters" to a previously shared story, itself associated with shame, forgiveness, and the hope of recovery.

At closer range, emotional support involves a more detailed disclosure of a story. The listener gently asks for a more detailed account, protects the recounting with an aura of safety, and shows in so many ways that the story has a home in the heart of the listener. At its most intimate – something well beyond the scope and appropriateness of most professional forms of care – emotional support involves knowing a person well.

OBSTACLES TO EMOTIONAL CARE

Emotional care is no less than the unseen floor, walls, and ceiling of social life itself. So it is worth understanding the obstacles to the acts of giving and receiving it. One obstacle is *appreciation starvation*. Care of an emotional sort often remains underappreciated. This is apparent when one looks at the various jobs – held mostly by women – in which emotional support plays an important role. Often the pay and status associated with caring work is not commensurate with the training it requires. Be they school teachers, social workers, nurses, nurses' aides, childcare workers, or elderly care attendants – none are among the most highly paid or honoured by our society. As a Montreal nurse complained to me, "I read in the paper that an actress who features in a daytime TV show was earning a million dollars per episode. At the same time, scores of nurses are quitting their jobs because of the low pay!" Money is a symbol of value in our society; thus low-paying jobs are often viewed as less important than high-paying ones. Comparing her fate to that of the movie star, the nurse felt, as she said, that "sometimes the care I give goes unseen, unrecognized, unappreciated." She then faces a certain "catch-22 of appreciation." Not getting it from the usual quarters (in pay, social status), she looks for appreciation from those around her, especially from those of higher status (doctors, for example). As she recounted, doctors are often painfully unattuned to both patients and nurses, and are held above any criticism they might receive for being so. Thus part of the emotional labour of the nurse involves suppressing her disappointment or exasperation at the absence of feedback for her hard work.

If the first obstacle reduces feedback on good emotional care, the second obstacle – *pressure to speed up* – makes it harder to actually offer such care. Restructuring and downsizing in the health care system, and the privatization of certain services, promotes a "for profit culture." This puts a premium on quantitative performance, which in turn leads to a redefinition of what care is. Health care providers feel pressured to handle more patients in a shorter amount of time. When I asked a woman who worked in an employee-assistance program how this "speed-up" influenced the way she provided emotional care, she replied, "I focus on the outlines of an employee's story and don't get into the details. It makes it harder for me to open my heart." She becomes less invitational in her tone of voice, more distant, more closed – either by becoming more speedy and time-conscious or by becoming less attuned. To some extent, she is "tuning out" those she's there to help.

To add insult to injury, many care workers who are being pressed to be more efficient absorb that stress – internalize it and cover it up – thus disguising the pressure they are under. To understand the social pressure they are putting on themselves, one would have to go back to its sources – the speed-up itself. In my studies, I found that part of a flight attendant's job description, for example, was to "enjoy the job." So when a speed-up occurred, part of her job, paradoxically, was to enjoy the speed-up.

A third strain on one's provision of emotional care – *displacements from caregiver to care recipient* – is only occasionally evident, and rarely recognized, which is why it is worth mentioning here. Many medical personnel who deal with the primary needs of patients (wash them, turn them in bed, provide and empty bed pans) suffer the indignities mentioned above but, in addition, find themselves low paid workers servicing high status clients. Their emotional labour consists not only of dealing with the absence of status and recognition for the care they give but also of dealing with their own understandable envy of those for whom they care. In the absence of efforts to counter envy, some workers may project ill feelings onto their privileged patients: "You're on vacation here," the worker may feel. "You get to sit there and have food brought to you while I have to work two jobs to make ends meet." I once interviewed a female doctor who had been hospitalized for an illness. Remarking on the nurse's aide, who she described as "unresponsive and surly," she said, "I got the feeling that she thought I was an idle, bon-bon eating, upper-class housewife, the kind of woman her mother had worked for as a maid, and this was an opportunity for her to put me in my place." An understandable feeling becomes an obstacle to emotional care.

Displacement also works the other way, creating a fourth obstacle – *displacements from the family of the patient to the care provider.* The families of patients, that is, can displace feelings onto the caregiver; only here the relevant feeling is not envy but guilt. Over the past thirty years in the US, the proportion of women working outside of the home has risen from one-third to two-thirds. Sixty-five per cent of mothers with children aged one to five are now members of the workforce. The proportion of part-time work among women has not increased in that period. In addition, from the 1990s on, work hours have been on the rise. There are more women and mothers on the work-train, and the train is going faster. On the other hand, in the United States, spending on social programs is being reduced, so both library hours and after-school recreation programs are being shortened. Furthermore, families are being told by governments, "We are going to outsource care to the family." Patients are being sent home sooner after major operations, with the idea that someone at home will take care of them. But who is at home to provide the care? Less and less is it mom and dad, and often grandma and the siblings are at work as well.

The combination of these trends has created a care deficit. The strain of this care deficit, in turn, generates a certain amount of guilt – particularly among women, the traditional caregivers at home. As family members of patients, they may inadvertently displace their guilt onto hospital staff via a rain of criticisms of the care the patient receives.

In an interview a physician told me: "I think a lot of the families of geriatric patients feel guilty, especially the more educated ones, and that will make them very demanding of the physician." Hospital personnel might be faced with a family member calling to insist that she/he be informed daily of any change in the diet or drugs being given to an elderly parent. Then another member of the same family will call to check up on something else. Eventually, the patient's chart will have an additional entry: "Difficult family." Behind the entry "difficult family" may lurk displaced guilt.

Each obstacle to the delivery of emotional care has a deep social root that calls, in turn, for deep social solutions. The solution to displaced envy, for example, lies in improving opportunities for hospital orderlies and generally in reducing the enormous and expanding social class gap within the wider society. The solution to displaced guilt is to reduce demands on working families. In the meantime, the emotional labour of the care worker includes the task of addressing the "referred pain" of larger social strains as it shows up in face-to-face interactions between caregiver and receiver. Among other things, the caregiver has to deal with the secondary consequences of long range problems.

WHO TAKES CARE OF THE CAREGIVERS? THE BUSMAN'S HOLIDAY

How do nurses cope with all of these obstacles and nonetheless provide emotional care? Who do *they* go to for care? I recently asked one nurse, "Do you go to your husband when you're frustrated, have encountered difficulties at work, or are upset?" Her husband worked long hours and was not interested in the details of her hard day. "Just give me the headlines," he told her. Her parents were unhelpfully anxious about her, so she didn't take her worries to her parents for fear of making them more anxious. One sibling lived in another town, and she was estranged from the other. The priest at the local church was not a viable source of support, and there was no time to participate in community activities that might provide a source of people to talk to. Nor were formal care-oriented organizations – such as a company-sponsored counsellor – part of her social world. Between work, home, children, and elderly parents, this nurse just could not find time for herself.

Instead, she sought care from *other nurses*, including the nurse with whom she daily drove home. "Sometimes I'm so upset," she told me, "I give my friend (the fellow nurse) the keys, saying, 'You drive while I talk.'" Like the busman who goes on a driving holiday, the nurse may do off duty what she does on duty – provide emotional care.

To conclude, one basic form of "emotional care" is tuning into the experience of another. It takes a subtle and vital form of emotional labour to stay attuned, especially in light of the many obstacles, internal and external, to the giving and receiving of care. All relationships – and the social worlds built upon them – depend on many small, hard-won moments of emotional attunement. Those who attune themselves to others need someone tuned into them. And it is often true that behind every great caregiver is another great caregiver.

6

Patient Emotions in a Clinical Context: Coping with Anxiety and Depression and Other Negative Emotions

GILBERT PINARD

Emotions impact on all aspects of people's health care: the rapidity with which they consult, the ease with which they speak of symptoms, their adherence to treatment regimens, their satisfaction with their interactions with the health care system, and, indeed, the very disorders they experience. In this chapter, I will address, from a clinical perspective, some of these considerations that I have encountered not only as a psychiatric consultant in a first-line community clinic, but also as a teacher and researcher in a university hospital clinic specialized in cognitive behavioural therapy. This approach highlights the links between cognition, emotions, and consequent behaviours. Hence the subject matter at hand is what patients think about themselves and their health, their care givers, and the health system, and what their emotions are about these appraisals.

As an example, a patient seen recently viewed his depression as an indication that he was a weak person and thought that antidepressants were addictive. He felt threatened and devalued by the prescription of medication and thus was non-compliant. Because he was ashamed to talk of his disorder with his family, people closest to him were unaware of this situation. Consequently, they were of little help and support. In general, 50 to 60 per cent of patients do not take their medications as prescribed, if at all.

DEFINING EMOTIONS

One of the first questions to be addressed is: "Do we know what our patients are referring to when they talk to us about their emotions?"

Figure 1
Psychiatrist and patient disagreement on primary affect

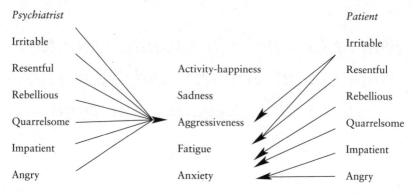

Source: Copyright 1974 Karger AG. Adapted, with permission of the publisher, from G. Pinard and and L. Tétreault, "Concerning semantic problems in psychological evaluation," *Modern Problems of Pharmacopsychiatry* 7 (1974): 13.

When using adjective lists to describe affects in depression, patients and psychiatrists do not necessarily agree. This is illustrated in Figure 1. The six adjectives shown are, for the psychiatrist, associated with "aggressiveness," while patients primarily associate these adjectives with "anxiety" (Pinard and Tétreault 1974).

There are also important cultural differences. Asian and Middle Eastern patients often present with physical symptoms rather than complain about emotional distress. They very rarely speak of "feeling blue or depressed" (Pinard 1987). What is meant by the very word "depression" is also important to clarify. Do we mean the emotion itself, the syndrome, or the disorders that bear the name?

THE EFFECTS OF EMOTIONS
ON HEALTH BEHAVIOURS

The mere expression of emotions has an impact on health behaviours. Consider alexithymia, which is the incapacity to talk of emotions. A recent study showed that individuals scoring high on scales measuring this construct have more maladaptive health habits such as bad nutrition, smoking, a sedentary life, and a higher propensity for substance abuse (Helmers and Mente 1999). What then is the connection between the expression of emotion and pathology?

There is also the whole area of emotions concerning consultation and disclosure. In our own research clinic, patients with severe obsessive compulsive disorder (OCD) take an average of 10.4 years before they first consult. I am not referring to patients with mild cases but with severe dysfunctions. For example, we had a patient who, for years, was so afraid of contamination that he would spend hours everyday washing. He lived secluded in his basement with all the furniture covered with plastic bags and ordered out for frozen foods, regarding them as less likely to be infected. This person was so ashamed that it was years before he dared to speak to someone about his condition.

We have found that patients suffering from social anxiety also take more than ten years to consult. Worse, many do not consult at all. The fear of disease is also an emotion that impacts on consultation. A patient recently revealed that he had experienced great difficulty urinating for several months. He had not consulted because he dreaded a diagnosis of prostate cancer. As for the elderly, some studies show that they do not refuse mental health counselling when offered, but the referral rate is low. This is true not only of the elderly living alone, but also of those living with a spouse or a friend. Only nursing home residency and referral by a physician improves attendance at therapy sessions (Mosher-Ashley 1995).

Even more troubling is another recent study on physical health care. The authors found that the delay in seeking treatment for heart attack symptoms ranged from 2 to 6.5 hours. This is a disturbing reality since it has been proven that an intervention within the first hour optimizes treatment (Dracup, Moser, Eisenberg, Meischke, Alonzo, and Braslow 1995). Emotions, including fear, also impact on preventive measures such as breast examinations. A study has shown that women at high risk examine themselves more often if they are more anxious; some, on the other hand, do not palpate for fear of finding something (Brain, Norman, Gray, and Mansel 1999). A generalized anxiety disorder patient of mine never touched her breasts and had to be more or less dragged to her physician even though she had a loaded family history and some signs of problems. She simply did not want to find out. We also had an OCD patient in the clinic who repeatedly examined herself several hours a day; it was her belief that, if ever she developed cancer and had not done the proper palpation, she would be responsible for her illness.

These few examples clearly indicate that there is considerable interference from emotions and beliefs at the very point of the patients' entry into the health care system. They show how crucial it is to pursue research into coping mechanisms (such as denial) and self-concept variables (such as helplessness), as well as into socio-economic factors, so as to develop ways of promoting survival behaviours, a crucial one being, obviously, simply to consult a physician.

THE EFFECTS OF MOOD
ON MEDICAL CONDITIONS

There is considerable literature on the effects of mood on pathophysiology and medical conditions. One of the shibboleths in the lay "self-help" press is the idea that we should "let it all hang out" and "speak our deep seated anger." The results of an atherosclerosis risk study entitled "Anger Proneness Predicts Coronary Heart Disease" (Williams, Paton, Siegler, Eigenbrodt, Nieto, and Tyroler 2000) goes counter to that idea. When the nearly 13,000 patients enrolled in the study were assessed using the Spielberger Trait Anger scale, it was found that high trait anger was associated with a twofold increased risk of coronary heart disease and a threefold increased risk of "hard events" in normotensives. This study was all the more interesting because it was prospective.

In 1999 at the Seventieth American Heart Association meeting, data were presented showing that men who get angry are twice as likely to have a stroke as those who are better at diffusing anger (Everson 1997). The study also showed that "suppressing anger" was likewise not a great strategy because of increased risk of high blood pressure. The conclusion is that "diffusing" anger through different adaptive coping techniques is the way to approach problems. For this study, the social behaviour of over 2,000 men was examined over a seven-year period, taking into account life habits as well as body mass, medication, diabetes, etc. Not only do outright outbursts of anger seem to be damaging, but so does irritability; as "irritability" and "dominance" increase, so do the odds of coronary heart disease (Siegman, Townsend, Civelek, and Blumenthal 2000). Another study (Stoll, Hamann, Mangold, Huf, and Winterhoff-Spurk 1999) reports that when shown violent scenes, men have an increase in middle cerebral artery blood pressure. Fortunately, the response is normotensive when the subjects are shown erotic scenes!

MENTAL DISORDERS AS THEY RELATE
TO MEDICAL CONDITIONS

Many studies have linked mental disorders and medical conditions. In a huge multicultural study published in the *Journal of the American Medical Association*, it was found that psychopathology was consistently associated with greater disability than was physical illness, even when controlling for physical illness. Severity of impairment grew with severity of mental illness; the disability was greatest in the case of major depression, panic disorder, and generalized anxiety disorder. These results held up in different cultural settings (Ormel, VonKorff, Ustun, Pini, Korten, and Oldehinkel 1994).

Table 1
Ten leading causes of disability-adjusted life years (DALY)

Rank	Disease or injury	DALYs Males ('000)	DALYs Females ('000)	DALYs Total ('000)
1	Unipolar major depression	15,554	27,651	42,972
2	Tuberculosis	15,321	8,736	19,673
3	Road traffic accidents	13,096	7,508	19,625
4	Alcohol use	11,040	7,095	14,848
5	Self-inflicted injuries	10,937	6,453	16,645
6	Bipolar disorder	7,899	6,419	13,189
7	War	7,550	5,964	13,134
8	Violence	6,786	5,896	12,955
9	Schizophrenia	6,646	5,367	12,242
10	Iron deficiency	5,098	5,235	12,511

Source: Copyright 1996 World Health Organization. Reprinted, with permission of the publisher, from C.J. Murray and A.D. Lopez, "The global burden of disease in 1990: Final results and their sensitivity to alternative epidemiological perspectives, discount rates, age weights and disability weights," in C.J. Murray and A.D. Lopez, eds, *The Global Burden of Disease: A Comprehensive Assessment of Mortality and Disability from Diseases, Injuries, and Risk Factors in 1990 and Projected to 2020*, vol. 1 (Cambridge, Mass.: Harvard School of Public Health, on behalf of the World Health Organization and the World Bank, distributed by Harvard University Press, 1996), 270.

I will pursue the connection between mental disorder and medical conditions more closely by focusing on depression and anxiety, their epidemiology and social impact, and their relation with physical disorders. In a national comorbidity survey, the twelve-month prevalence for any anxiety disorder was 19.3%; depression was at 11.3%, as were addictive disorders. Within the mood disorders, the breakdowns were: major depression at 10.3%, dysthymia at 2.5%, and mania at 1.3% (Kessler, McGonagle, Zhao, Nelson, Hughes, Eshleman, Wittchen, and Kendler 1996). As for the ten leading causes of disability-adjusted life years (DALY), as measured in 1996, unipolar depression ranked number one, twice as high as either tuberculosis or road traffic accidents, and almost three times higher than alcohol use (Murray and Lopez 1996)

As for the costs to the workplace, it has been determined that, in the US, depression alone costs an astounding 33 billion US dollars: $25 billion in absenteeism and $8 billion in lost productivity (Greenberg, Kessler, Nells, Finkelstien, and Berndt 1996). With such a prevalence of depression and anxiety, and their damage to people's lives, why are so many of those suffering from them not in treatment? It would seem people continue to doubt efficacy, ignore the urgency to treat, or believe that it is important to their self-image that they solve the problem on their own. This remains the case despite forty years of effective medications and constant refinements of the pharmacology of antidepressants and twenty years of research and publications about the effective psychotherapies for depression and anxiety disorders.

DEPRESSION AND MEDICAL ILLNESS

The increased odds ratio of getting a myocardial infarction (MI) if a history of depression is present is enormous: 4.5 for major depression and 2.0 for dysthymia. In May 2000 the National Health and Nutrition Examination Survey reported on a ten-year follow up of over 5,000 women and 3,000 men first assessed between 1982 and 1984. The general rate of depression was more than 17 per cent, which is typical of epidemiological data. Both men and women were at an over 70 per cent increased risk of coronary heart disease if they had been depressed. Men also had the distinction of an increased risk of death ratio of 2.4 (Ferketich, Schwartzbaum, Frid, and Moeschberger 2000).

Another study, conducted at the Montreal Heart Institute, found that over 30 per cent of patients with coronary artery disease suffer from depression (Frasure-Smith, Lespérance, and Talajic 1993). Most troubling is the odds ratio of 3.6 for the impact of depression on the mortality rate, as can be seen in Figure 2.

The prognostic impact of depression is about as large as, and independent of, other major prognostic factors. Anxiety also correlates with increased risk of MI and seems somewhat independent of "history of depression" or of "depression at the time of the event." In addition, a separate study has documented the impact of depression on angina. In a five-year prospective study, 200 patients of a Health Maintenance Organization (HMO) were evaluated. Initial depression scores correlated with severity of angina after five years (frequency, stability of angina), as well as with work limitations, perception of the·disease, and satisfaction with the treatment. In strokes, the evidence is that depression actually precedes it and has the same epidemiology as MIs afterwards (Sullivan, LaCroix, Russo, Swords, Sornson, and Katon 1999).

In sum, depression impacts both on peoples' health and on the health system. It was found that the added costs to the system increase more than 40 per cent if the patient who has a coronary heart disease also suffers from depression. Despite the links between depression and heart conditions, cardiac patients do not make it easy to diagnose depression. They have a tendency to normalize their distress, to speak of tiredness, and to predictably report more anxiety and worrying than sadness.

Figure 2
Major depression post MI: Impact on eighteen-month survival

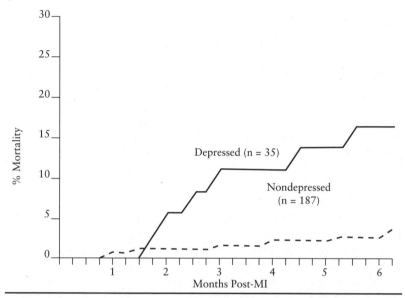

Cumulative mortality for depressed and nondepressed patients. MI indicates myocardial infarction.

Source: Copyright 1994 American Medical Association. Reprinted, with permission of the publisher, from N. Frasure-Smith, F. Lespérance, and M. Talajic, "Depression following myocardial infarction: Impact on 6-month survival," *Journal of the American Medical Association* 270 (1994): 1,821.

Yet this depression is treatable, and, with minimal interventions, the survival rate is improved (Lespérance and Frasure-Smith 2000).

IMPACT OF EMOTIONS ON THE QUALITY OF LIFE

Mendlowicz and Stein (2000) report that, overall, major depression has a greater impact on "quality of life" than do all anxiety disorders combined. However, the domains of quality affected are similar. Perception of mental functioning is reduced in both groups by close to 40 per cent, but depressives also see themselves as physically sicker than "normals." Role performance – i.e., social and emotional functioning – is similarly lowered by at least 30 per cent in patients with anxiety and depressive disorders (Mendlowicz and Stein 2000).

Though many therapeutic strategies, such as medications and cognitive behavioural therapy (CBT), can improve people's conditions, some authors have explored the barriers to treatment, be they identification of the problem, reluctance to seek help, poor compliance, or uncertainty about which treatment paradigm is best. For example, it has been reported that patients suffering from severe social anxiety, which impacts on both their social and work functioning, are reluctant to consult even when they realize they have a problem. Beyond the financial constraints and finding out where to go, the issue of what people will think of them and what people will say to them at work becomes central in their decision making about treatment (Olfson, Guardino, Struening, and Schneier 2000).

EMOTIONS AND CAREGIVERS

The "*virage ambulatoire*" in the Quebec health care system (the centring of care in the community, rather than in the hospital environment) has meant that many caregiver roles have been handed over to spouses and other family members. Such a transfer of responsibility needs to be accompanied by a transfer of information concerning coping strategies. These caregivers need to learn not only to problem-solve, but also to cope with their own emotions in this context. In psychiatry for example, we now see older parents caring for their agitated or suicidal adult children. These parents often feel overwhelmed and express a sense of helplessness. They are often afraid physically, unknowledgeable medically, and unprepared emotionally for these added responsibilities. Nursing journals report on how both nurses and spouses need to develop new strategies for home care (O'Brien 1993).

As for the caregivers in hospitals, some of them are dealing with new infectious diseases such as AIDS, which at times makes them feel vulnerable and affects both their emotions and behaviours. In caring for people with HIV, for instance, worry and discomfort are especially strong in nurses involved in "invasive contacts." Avoidance of certain tasks or, indeed, certain types of patients, as well as stress related absences, need to be monitored and remedied (Dworkin, Albrecht, and Cooksey 1991).

COPING WITH EMOTIONS

Finally we come to coping with emotions and the strategies needed for patients, relatives, and, indeed, staff. I will be looking at coping from a clinician's point of view and in a cognitive therapy practitioner's context. Cognitive therapy has focused on what people make of a situation. It targets their assumptions and beliefs about a specific event and their concepts of self and the world. Also, the emotional context interacts with these cognitions and with what individuals bring to this context – i.e., their behavioural inclinations, such as flight, fight, or freeze in fearful situations; or isolation, withdrawal, or inactivity when suffering from depression. Hence the therapist will look at these appraisals with the patient and identify the patient's emotional state and behavioural repertoire, collaborating with the patient in order to establish better modes of adaptation. Much literature on locus of control and attribution fits in neatly with the CBT clinical concepts. I will review but a few examples that demonstrate the impact of these concepts on health care, health promoting behaviours, and compliance.

Studies have shown that people with an internal locus of control have a greater sense of mastery, or competence. Those reliant on external controls, on the other hand, have a tendency to feel helpless. They have greater difficulty in trying to stop smoking, have a higher attrition rate in exercise programs, and, in general, are less informed about health related issues (Lefcourt and Davidson-Katz 1991). Taking the example of MI patients, those with an internal locus of control were less depressed and more cooperative while in intensive care and had shorter stays in hospital. Those with external controls, by comparison, felt more helpless when undergoing serious surgical interventions and were consequently more depressed.

Concerning psychiatric disorders, patients who attribute positive outcomes to externals and negative results to themselves have a greater sense of depression and lower expectancies regarding positive outcomes of treatment. Not only do depressed individuals have a greater sense that success is attributable to external causes and failure attributable to themselves, but they also believe this pattern to be stable over time and generalize it to many if not all situations. This "pessimistic" explanatory style (Burns and Seligman 1991) was found to predict poorer health thirty-five years later (Peterson, Seligman, and Vaillant 1988).

Turning to coping, many have written about coping as a mediator of emotion. One analysis (Folkman and Lazarus 1988) divides coping strategies into two focuses: problem solving (which includes planning and confronting strategies) and emotion (which includes strategies such as distancing, self-control, and escape/avoidance). Seeking social support, for example, can be seen not only as partly problem solving focused, if it involves seeking information, but also as partly emotion focused, if it is done to find a sympathetic ear. To determine if coping mediates emotion, this analysis looked at what happens in stressful situations. It was found that "planful" problem solving is associated with an improved emotional state, whereas "confronting" leads to worsened emotional states – which corroborates the data indicating that "getting it off your chest" is not an efficient strategy. People with high depression scores used anger more than those with low scores. One would have to look more at assertiveness as opposed to the expression of anger and approach therapeutic strategies accordingly. Also of interest is that emotion-focused approaches seem short-lived. Distancing, either physically or mentally, while initially effective, leads to a worsened emotional state. This is particularly fascinating in the light of OCD patients who feel initially reassured by avoidance of situations that trigger their fears but eventually start the rituals all over again ... and again ...

In Figure 3 one can see where a clinician can intervene and apply some CBT principles to modify the appraisals and resultant emotions.

Figure 3
Coping as a mediator of emotion

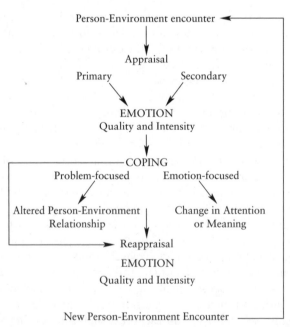

CONCLUSION

Emotions affect people's health, their quality of life, and their inter-actions with the health care system. Emotions such as depression and anxiety have a direct impact on some physiological processes, contrib-ute to the development of some disorders – supposedly both physical and mental (as if they can be separated by a hermetic barrier) – and/or greatly complicate the evolution of these disorders.

Emotions and appraisals bias the way patients seek help or not, whether they consult a physician, what they reveal and to whom, and how they collaborate in their treatment, taking or not taking respon-sibility for it. They also dictate, to some degree, how caregivers – whether they are professionals (nurses, social workers, psychologists, or physicians) or part of the patient's social network (family, friends, or neighbours) – interact with patients.

7

Patient Emotions and the "Engineering" of Provider Responses for More Effective Care

LAURETTE DUBÉ

Positive and negative emotions are feeling states that signal the occurrence of events that are relevant to important goals, motivating those who feel them to act in a certain manner and others to respond in a given way. Most of the time, episodes of illness are emotionally charged events, and ideally patients want professionals to consider their emotions when providing health care. Unfortunately, the full and systematic integration of patient emotions into the design and everyday delivery of health services seems to be a luxury that societies cannot afford given the exclusive focus on operational efficiency in the recent restructuring of health care in most modern countries. Moreover, there is also a popular belief that emotions may be so personal and idiosyncratic that they cannot (some would even say should not) be measured and systematically built into the design and management of health services.

In this chapter, I will first argue that, as we enter an era of chronic diseases with an aging clientele, the effectiveness of health services may be as closely tied to the providers' abilities to design and manage interactions with patients that take into account their emotional states during each care episode as it is to the provision of adequate biomedical care and information. I will then review two basic approaches to the measure of everyday emotions and present empirical findings from research that myself and other researchers from consumer and social psychology have been conducting on emotions in various contexts, including but not limited to the health domain. Finally, I will use some of the recent and ongoing research I have been doing with collaborators to illustrate what I mean by the "engineering" of providers' responses to patient emotions. As you will see, it has nothing to do with the "canned" or "mechanistic" stereotype that usually comes to mind.

"Engineering" consists of the mindful design and management of provider responses to patient emotions in a way that creates the most positive outcomes. The recent development of the "engineering" of provider responses to client emotions comes from the area of services marketing management (Arnould and Price 1993; Dubé and Morgan 1996b, 1998a). In commercial and non-commercial service industries, the engineering of provider responses to client emotions is important because what is being "produced" has an intrinsic human component, and, given that it is produced at the same time as it is consumed, post-hoc quality controls are relatively useless (Dubé, Johnson, and Renaghan 1999). Therefore, upfront planning of the human aspects of service quality may very well be necessary in order to prevent the client's emotions from interfering with operational efficiency while, at the same time, ensuring better quality for the client.

ON THE NEED TO CONSIDER EVERYDAY PATIENT EMOTIONS

Until now, formal consideration of patient emotions in the delivery of care has consisted primarily of psychotherapeutic interventions designed to help patients cope with negative emotions experienced at a clinical level either in the course of severe diseases or in highly stressful medical interventions or diagnostic procedures (for a review, see Dubé et al. 2002). Consideration of patient emotions in the everyday delivery of care is also implicitly built into the "art of care" that was part of Hippocrates' medical ethics and that, ever since, has been at the core of professional ethics and the socialization process for all health providers. Emotion is also an intrinsic component of the generally accepted biopsychosocial model of health (Engel 1977). Such general consideration of everyday emotions and other more human aspects of care may once have been sufficient for health care consisting primarily of acute interventions since many of the health outcomes in the acute setting are driven by the efficacy of the medical or surgical intervention. But this is no longer the case.

As we enter an era dominated by more chronic diseases within an aging population and by an increased reliance on community-based actions, the effective management of patient emotions may become just as central to quality of care as is the effectiveness of acute biomedical interventions. My argument is twofold. First, emotions are powerful drivers of everyday behaviour for everybody, and this is particularly the case for older individuals, who are the primary targets of chronic diseases. There is robust evidence that with increasing age, emotions may become more powerful than rational consideration of knowledge in motivating one to act (Carstensen and Turk-Charles 1994; Gross, Carstensen, Tsai, Skorpen, and Hsu 1997). Second, whereas some facets of emotions may evolve advantageously with aging, others don't, and these may pose challenges to one's health management. Research shows that the healthy elderly are more vulnerable than the healthy young to the adverse effects of negative emotional states on memory processes (Backman and Molander 1986; Deptula, Singh, and Pomara 1993). Memory becomes critical to the performance of appropriate health-maintaining or health-restoring behaviours when these behaviours are performed by the patient and/ or people in his or her social environment, which is increasingly the case with an aging clientele susceptible to chronic diseases. Thus, for the provider, having a more in-depth understanding of patient emotions and taking them into consideration in the design and delivery of health care may be more of a necessity than a luxury, even within a context of limited resources.

What I present next should demonstrate that it is possible to theoretically predict and empirically test not only the nature of the everyday emotions patients may feel in the context of receiving health care, but also their sensitivity to what happens over the course of the service process and the subsequent impact on various outcomes. In some respects, I will offer you seeds for a quantitative, "evidence-based" approach to the emotional aspects of health care akin to the approach that now prevails in the bioclinical domain. Even though the richness of human nature reflected in any emotion could never be reduced to its quantitative expression, such an approach may be necessary if emotions and the other more human aspects of care are to be put on the strategic and financial agenda for the design and management of health care in the future.

THE NATURE AND MEASURE
OF PATIENT EVERYDAY EMOTIONS

The term "patient everyday emotions" is used to specify that we are not concerned with negative emotions experienced at a clinical level but with positive and negative emotions as they naturally arise in the course of everyday life, including instances in which everyday life is tinted by sickness episodes. In the literature, the nature of everyday emotions has been conceptualized in two ways – i.e., as basic affective dimensions and as specific emotional states not reducible to basic dimensions.

Basic Affective Dimensions of Emotions

As basic affective dimensions, emotions are generally measured on multi-item, self-report scales in which a person indicates the intensity and/or frequency with which he/she experiences a set of emotional states like joy, happiness, fear, anxiety, etc. These self-reports of emotions are then submitted to data reduction techniques to extract basic affective dimensions like general positive and negative affects (Watson, Clark, and Tellegen 1988). Typically, basic affective dimensions are then used as predictors of a diversity of judgments and behaviours, and their moderators are investigated. For instance, research has shown that positive and negative affects are associated with the experience and reporting of different physical symptoms (e.g., Diefenbach, Leventhal, Leventhal, and Patrick-Miller 1996). We can monitor the change over time in the intensity with which these affects are experienced (e.g., Marco and Suls 1993). The influence of individual characteristics like gender (e.g., Dubé and Morgan 1998a) and chronic negative affectivity (Marco and Suls 1993) on the intensity and pattern of change in the basic positive and negative affects have also been recognized.

Research has shown that the basic negative affect dimension can be differentiated further as a function of the source from which negative feelings arise (Weiner 1985). In a field study conducted with adult patients in an acute care facility, we (Dubé, Bélanger, and Trudeau 1996a) found that in reporting, upon departure, the emotions they experienced during their stay, patients differentiated their negative emotions on the basis of whether they could attribute them to the naturally aversive quality of hospitalization (e.g., anxious, worried, and depressed feelings) or to the actions of the health care providers (e.g., frustrated, angry, feeling of being treated like a number). Albeit less salient in the structure of patient emotions, we also found a self-attributed negative affect dimension that grouped emotions like shame and guilt. We found, which is somewhat intriguing in this study, that the situation-attributed negative emotions were positively linked with patient satisfaction – i.e., the more the patients retrospectively reported having experienced situation-attributed emotions like anxiety and depressed feelings, the more satisfied they declared having been with the health services they had received. Not surprisingly, for other-attributed negative emotions like anger and frustration, we found, as expected, a strong and inverse relationship with satisfaction.

The above findings of a positive link between the patient's experience of situation-attributed negative emotions were unusual at the time since it had been traditionally believed that the emotions one experienced during the service process had valence-congruent effects on evaluative judgments, such as satisfaction – i.e., that negative emotions induced negative evaluations and that the converse was true for positive emotions (see Oliver 1997 for a review). We, and others, have since documented redundant findings of a positive relationship between situation-attributed negative emotions and satisfaction with other heath care services (Brown and Kirmani 1999; Dubé and Menon 1998b). What were the factors underlying the positive relationship between anxiety and satisfaction? There were many.

A positive relationship between situation-attributed negative emotions and satisfaction might have resulted from a given level of health services being perceived as positive by mere comparison with one's negative emotional states prior to receiving these services. If this had been the case, however, the relationship between emotions and satisfaction should have been the same across all negative affective dimensions. This was not the case. A second explanation for the positive relationship between negative situation-attributed emotions and satisfaction could be that providers are able to pick up cues from patient emotions and use these to fine-tune the quality of care in a way that helps patients to deal successfully with their negative feelings, thereby inducing higher satisfaction. In a follow-up study conducted in a service industry other than health, although we again observed the positive relationship between situation-attributed negative emotions and client satisfaction, when controlling for provider response, this relationship became insignificant (Dubé, Jedidi, and Menon 1997). This result is consistent with the interpersonal explanation. However, to delve more rigorously into the proposed interpersonal dynamics requires a more detailed understanding of emotional episodes than that provided by numerical ratings of emotions reduced to basic dimensions. Such a more complex approach to emotions is presented next.

Multicomponent Approach to Specific Emotions

As an alternative to basic affective dimensions, emotions are also viewed as specific feeling states, whose richness can only be captured by a more complex representation of these episodes. This view and its numerous versions have received a diversity of labels in the literature (e.g., Izard 1977; Parkinson 1995; Sherer 1984; Shaver, Schwartz, Kirson, and O'Connor 1987). We will group these labels under the umbrella of the multicomponent approach to emotions. According to this perspective, emotions are organized response patterns comprising cognitive, experiential, physiological, expressive, behavioural and interpersonal components. Each of these components has a specific purpose and operates in a temporal and logical sequence to enable the interface between an individual and the environment. Whereas quantitative self-reports have sometimes been used (e.g., Izard 1977), the bulk of research in the multicomponent approach to emotions has tapped into the layperson's mental representations of emotional episodes arising from repeated experiences, thereby eliciting scripts of specific emotional episodes (e.g., anger, anxiety, joy, etc.).

Scripts of emotional episodes are typically elicited by semistructured interviews or questionnaires in which a person is asked to recollect an emotional episode of a specific type, guided by a series of prompts that correspond to the various script components. The four emotion components that capture most of the complexity of emotional episodes and the prompts used to elicit these are: (1) *appraisal of the circumstances* in which an emotion arose (what happened, when, why, in what context?); (2) *subjective experience and expression* (how did it feel, what did you do, what did you say, etc.?); (3) *action/coping tendencies* (how did you react to and/or deal with the emotion? e.g., asked someone for reassurance); (4) *expected and observed interpersonal responses* (how did you expect others to respond to your emotional expression? e.g., expected reassurance; how did they respond? e.g., ignored me).

Scripts are constructed from a sample of respondents' most frequent answers to the prompts for each component. Over the years, the literature has provided fairly reliable generic representations in daily-life settings of specific emotions like anxiety, anger, sadness, joy, etc. Table 1 presents the script for emotional episodes of anxiety and anger. Here, we will underscore some key similarities and differences between the two specific emotions. Whereas both anxiety and anger arise when an environmental stimuli is appraised as being incongruent with one's goals, the *appraisal* dimensions of certainty, control, and agency distinguish the two types of emotional episodes (Smith and Ellsworth 1985). Anxiety generally arises from events perceived as being uncertain and attributable only to uncontrollable circumstances, in the face of which one feels powerless. In contrast, anger stems from appraisals indicating that one is relatively certain of what happened and is associated with the attribution of blame to others and with a sense of individual control and power. In terms of *subjective experience and expression*, both emotions are unpleasant feelings entailing high arousal, but they differ in their expression, with anger translating into much more aggressive expressions than anxiety.

In the context of *action/coping tendencies,* the terminologies used in the various multicomponent approaches to emotions vary tremendously. In Table 1, we organized the forms taken by the behavioural response component on the basis of Folkman and Lazarus's well-known model

Table 1
Generic scripts of emotional episodes of anxiety and anger

	Anxiety	Anger
Appraisals	Sudden, unpleasant, highly relevant, situational attribution, uncertainty, low control, low power	Unpleasant, highly relevant, other attribution, certainty, high control, high power
Experience/ expression	Fear, unpleasant high arousal, perspiring, heart pounding, shaking, eyes darting	Tense, unpleasant high arousal, clenched fists, threatening frowning, gritting teeth
Action/coping tendencies	Emotion-focused responses: seeking reassurance and distancing	Problem-focused responses: planful problem solving, confrontation/attack
Expected interpersonal responses	Emotional support strategies	Instrumental support strategies
Observed interpersonal responses	Emotional support strategies	No support/attack or ignore

of coping (Folkman and Lazarus 1985). In this model, behavioural responses to emotion-eliciting events can be of two types: emotion-focused and problem-focused. *Emotion-focused* responses are primarily directed at regulating the emotion rather than altering the person/ environment. *Problem-focused* responses refer to active attempts to attack and solve the problem. It is important to note that within each of these two broad types, response tendencies can invite others either to react positively to one's emotions or to push one away. Research indicates that anxiety episodes are associated with emotion-focused responses that can equally involve approach tendencies, such as affiliating more with others and seeking emotional aid, and avoidance tendencies, such as distancing oneself from the situation, a tendency that does not invite others' responses. Problem-focused responses and anxiety are generally not related in generic scripts elicited from daily-life settings. In contrast, anger is related primarily to problem-focused responses that attempt to change aspects of the individual/environment relationship, either by confrontive responses (being aggressive towards the perceived cause) or by planful problem solving (changing the perceived cause or facets of it).

Concerning *interpersonal responses* to one's emotions, we organized the forms that this component can take into two categories: emotional support and instrumental support. This builds on Thoits's (1986) demonstration that the coping strategies used by individuals in response to their own emotions are the same as those utilized by others in response to these emotions. Emotional support strategies refer to the demonstration of empathic understanding, reassurance, or other positive reactions without attempting to address the underlying event that gave rise to the emotion. Evidence indicates that anxious individuals generally expect others to provide emotional support strategies, an expectation that is usually met by others. For instance, Simpson, Rholes, and Nelligan (1992) found that as the level of anxiety and the tendency to seek emotional aid increased in women subjects, others displayed greater emotional support responses. Angry individuals, on the other hand, expect others to provide instrumental support, which others frequently fail to provide, oftentimes reacting with a similar level of anger (Palfai and Hart 1997). In fact, research suggests that anger may be the most contagious emotion (Tavris 1984).

Thus it seems that anxiety and anger – exemplars respectively of situation-attributed and other-attributed emotions in the studies cited earlier on the relationship between patient emotions and satisfaction – differ in the degree of match between the expected versus observed interpersonal responses to one's emotions. The provider's propensity to react in a manner perceived as appropriate by the client seems much higher in response to anxiety than it does in response to anger. It is possible that in the previous studies, it was the match between what anxious patients were expecting as an interpersonal response from the providers and what they actually received as an interpersonal response (i.e., providers offered emotional support to the patient) that contributed to patient satisfaction. In contrast, patients who were feeling angry might have been less likely to observe an interpersonal response from the providers that conformed to their expectations (i.e., patients expected instrumental support and received either no support or hostile, aggressive responses). This mismatch, in conjunction with appraisal of blame attribution, is likely to have induced the strong and reverse link between anger and patient satisfaction.

Although we do not yet have patient data to present in support of the above proposition, we observed in related work conducted in retail services (Menon and Dubé 1999b, 2000) that providers are indeed more likely to react to a client's episodes of anxiety in a way that leads to satisfaction than they are to episodes of anger. In fact, in the more recent of these two studies, we found that in more than seven cases out of ten, clients reported that the provider reacted to their anger in a way that did not conform to their expectations: Oftentimes the provider responded in an equally aggressive fashion or by ignoring them. In this study, we again found that the client's perception of the provider's response to negative emotions mediated their impact on satisfaction. Thus there is a real payoff in terms of outcomes in ensuring that providers give the most effective response to client emotions. Unfortunately, one cannot rely simply on everybody's goodwill to make this happen. Some mindful design and management is needed.

ENGINEERING PROVIDER RESPONSES TO PATIENT EMOTIONS

As mentioned at the outset of this chapter, the engineering of providers' responses to client emotions has been defined in the services marketing and management literature as the mindful design and management of the providers' responses to client emotions at any phase of the service consumption process. Such engineering induces positive outcomes like satisfaction and loyalty, which in the health domain translate into satisfaction and compliance. There are two equally important steps in the engineering of provider responses to patient emotions: the elicitation of *emotion scripts in context* and the *evidence-based validation* of the effectiveness of alternative provider response strategies in inducing positive outcomes.

Scripting Emotional Episodes in Context

Compared to the previously reported generic scripts that are primarily elicited in daily-life settings, the form taken by the script components of an emotional episode may differ in important ways when these are elicited in the context of purposeful exchanges such as those that occur in service industries like health care. Either because of explicit and implicit social roles and mutual obligations between the client and the provider or because of the level of service quality considered acceptable in given industries, incongruities between the client's action/coping tendencies when faced with a specific emotion and the provider's response are particularly critical. For instance, problem-focused responses to anxiety are generally not elicited in scripts derived from daily-life settings. However, we have found that in the context of retail services (Menon 1999a; Menon and Dubé 2000) and airline services (Menon and Dubé 2001), problem-focused responses to anxiety episodes are highly prevalent.

Moreover, in the context of airline services, which have exhibited an ever-increasing incidence of delays and service failures of all sorts (ACSI 2000), we (Menon and Dubé 2001) found that on certain occasions clients, even when they knew that providers were likely at the root of the event that had elicited their negative emotional responses, still reported the episode as being one dominated by anxiety, as they were unwilling to devote the potentially useless additional emotional energy needed to feel and show anger (Berkowitz 1993). In addition, the same clients reported that their most prevalent emotion-focused action/coping tendency was not one of seeking reassurance, as was found to be the case in the generic scripts, but rather most often one of distancing themselves from their emotions. In such a context, provider response strategies based on the provision of emotional support may have little impact on positive outcomes.

Thus the first step in engineering provider responses to patient emotions is to position the most critical emotional episodes along the continuum of care and to elicit scripts for these emotions in the specific context of care in which engineering is to be applied. Prompts similar to those presented earlier should be adjusted to the specific context of application. In addition, it is also critical, once a first version of a patient's emotion script is elicited, to elaborate upon this version, taking into consideration the unique parameters of each service environment in which the engineering of a provider's response to patient emotions is to be applied. For instance, it is necessary to identify and assess the impact of factors both individual (e.g., patient and provider characteristics) and organizational (e.g., institutional culture, staffing practices) that may influence the precise forms that patients' action/coping tendencies take as well as the expected and observed interpersonal responses. These data will result in a portfolio of provider responses to patient emotions that is comprehensive and realistic enough to warrant its systematic yet flexible application. The rich understanding that such scripts can give of patients' emotional experiences can then be used for employee training, as well as for quality specification and management.

Evidence-Based Effectiveness of Provider Responses to Patient Emotions

Can the effectiveness of alternative provider response strategies for coping with a specific type of emotional episode be measured and empirically tested in a valid and reliable way so that the most effective strategy, or a portfolio of these, becomes known as such and systematically used in day-to-day practice? This would require that the impact on various outcomes of various strategies for dealing with specific emotions be empirically demonstrated and, ultimately, that the causal relationship be submitted to experimental investigation. Although trials to test the efficacy of specific emotional and interpersonal care strategies are still scant, I am convinced that such research can be done and that it would have as many potential benefits as similar studies have had in supporting evidence-based biomedical practices. To support my position, I will first present a brief overview of an on-going longitudinal study on patient emotions, provider responses, and their combined contribution to outcomes. This correlational study, conducted with elderly patients in a mid-term health care facility, will be built upon at a later stage, using randomized clinical trials, to test the relative effectiveness of alternative provider response strategies or, for that matter, the effectiveness of any intervention at all. To predict what forms this research may take, I will report on a simulation-based experiment that tested the relative effectiveness of alternative provider response strategies to episodes of anger and anxiety in the context of airline services.

Correlational evidence. Figure 1 presents a schematic overview of the on-going longitudinal study in which we are examining, for each patient under observation, a sequence of care episodes (health services surrounding meals).

In the study patient participants provide self-reports of specific emotions prior to and after the care episodes, and also report on their satisfaction with the service received. We are examining four emotions: anger, anxiety, depression, and generally positive feelings. On-line observations of interpersonal behaviours and the objective assessment of the quality of food intake for each meal, as well as the assessment of admission-departure nutritional status, complement the patient's self-reports. Data are being collected for a large number of care episodes for each patient so that we will be able to link patient emotions prior to a care episode to the interpersonal responses that these emotions triggered from the providers. Providers' interpersonal behaviours are recorded in terms of the four poles of the well-known Interpersonal Circumplex model: dominance, agreeableness, submissiveness, and quarrelsomeness. Using multilevel modelling techniques, the observed provider's interpersonal responses are assessed in terms of their contribution to: (1) the monitoring of patient emotions (changes in emotional states over the course of the care episode); (2) patient satisfaction with the care episode as a whole; and (3) short-term (quality of food intake) and long-term (change in nutritional status between admission and departure) clinical outcomes. We are presently collecting data and thus cannot yet present detailed results. However, we are convinced that such empirical exploration of the relationship between patient emotions, the provider's response to these emotions, and the impact of this response on patient outcomes is a necessary step towards a "randomized clinical trial" approach to the engineering of providers' responses to patient emotions in a way that will create the most positive outcomes.

Figure 1
Overview of a longitudinal, correlational study of patient emotions, providers'
responses, and the impact on care outcome in a mid-term health care facility

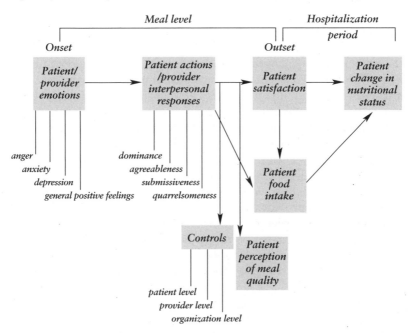

Experimental evidence. In the airline services experiment, we used written scenarios of an event that occurs frequently during air travel (waiting in line at the check-in counter) and a role playing methodology that enabled participants to easily and vividly relate to the air travel scenario described. In the scenario of the emotional episode, we first manipulated the cognitive appraisals – provider blame and uncontrollable circumstances – to evoke feelings of anger and anxiety respectively and then measured the subject's action/coping tendencies using the Ways of Coping Scale (Folkman, Lazarus, and Dunkel-Schetter 1986). Second, we manipulated the interpersonal response strategies performed by the provider. Participants were randomly assigned to one of four types of interpersonal reactions as provider strategies: emotional support (providing reassurance and empathy), instrumental support (active attempts to resolve the problem), mixed support (a combination of both emotional and instrumental support), and, as a control, no support. We then measured consumer satisfaction with the provider's response strategy.

Results showed that, regardless of the strategy, there was an increase in satisfaction when any response strategy was offered by the provider, compared to the control condition (no intervention). Across all emotional episodes, in the context of such purposeful exchanges as those that transpire in airline services, the provision of instrumental support was superior to that of emotional support. Results also showed that the adjunction of emotional support to instrumental support in the hybrid strategy had a significant incremental impact on satisfaction for a subset of clients only: it had no effect for those clients who tended to distance themselves from their emotions (predominantly those experiencing episodes of anxiety); it had a positive impact on clients whose action/coping tendencies were prevailingly confrontational (predominantly those experiencing episodes of anger). The results show that the engineering of provider responses to client emotions has a significant and positive impact on service outcomes and that, for this engineering to be effective, provider responses must be adapted to the value observed in the earlier components of the emotion script. Similar experimental tests, preferably using field intervention instead of scenario simulation, can be performed to determine the effectiveness of alternative provider response strategies to patient emotions.

CONCLUSION

The evidence I have presented suggests that everyday emotions experienced by patients in the process of receiving care can be measured and, with the assistance of the provider, managed and monitored in a way that positively influences the outcome of care. The question, then, is how to weave these human considerations into the design and management of health care in a more systematic fashion. We have first to develop scientific knowledge in these domains similar to that which abounds in the biomedical arena. This entails studying basic emotional and interpersonal processes that arise in the patient's experience and the provider's delivery of care as well as empirically validating the effectiveness of provider strategies for responding to patient emotions. Most importantly, such "normative" scripts have to be assimilated by the providers, in conjunction with their expertise and experience in the other domains of care, and they also have to be integrated with other aspects of care on a day-to-day basis. Finally, we have to measure and monitor their impact on organizational and clinical outcomes. Doing the above will help to ensure that emotions become an integrated component in health care research and practice. This formal integration of interpersonal emotion management into the delivery of care may entice and enable the patients to more effectively perform appropriate day-to-day behaviours themselves and to recruit the support they need for their health's management from their social network, from the community, or from formal health services.

8

Interpersonal Processes in the Patient-Physician Relationship

DEBRA L. ROTER

As I reflect on the current state of the patient-physician relationship, Norman Rockwell's portrait of the family doctor examining a little girl's doll springs to mind. It is an iconic reflection of a long-lost era when doctor-patient relationships were intimate, humane, thoughtful, engaging, and sensitive. In this portrait, the little girl is looking straight at the doctor, but his eyes are averted in concentration while listening to the stethoscope placed on the doll's heart. Closer inspection of the image reveals something amiss: the posture of deep concentration, with eyes averted, is one in which communication has been supplanted by technology. As noted by Shorter (1985) in his history of doctors and patients, the technological transformation of medicine in the last century was fundamental in redirecting medical inquiry from the person of the patient to the biochemical and pathophysiology of the patient. It was not coincidental that the practice of interviewing patients using a written outline designed around a series of yes-no hypothesis-testing questions replaced unstructured medical histories at this point in the history of medicine. As a result, the doctor lost the face-to-face contact that could provide insight into the patient's emotional, rather than merely physical, well-being.

This chapter has two objectives. First, I explore the interplay between the technical and emotional dimensions of health care. I do so by looking at the theoretical and philosophic basis defining the therapeutic relationship. Second, I explore the role of gender in shaping the expression of the therapeutic relationship. I include a brief summary of a meta-analysis of the literature describing the effects of physician gender on communication. That analysis is of interest because it highlights some of the interpersonal processes at play in establishing, maintaining, and shaping the doctor-patient relationship.

My thesis is threefold. First, I see the quality of the interactive process as being critical to the establishment of a therapeutic relationship; the quality of the doctor-patient dialogue reflects the nature of the relationship. Second, though patient sociodemographic characteristics, health status, health system speciality, and site variables all contribute to variations in the medical interaction and in the medical dialogue, physician variables consistently show significant independent effects. Dana Safran's chapter similarly suggests that doctor level variables affect study results more than site and practice characteristics. Finally, though gender is not the only significant physician-specific variable one might study, it is an important one and among the few that have been studied in any detail. Physician gender partly defines the therapeutic relationship, shaping it through gender-linked communication styles.

THE THEORETICAL AND PHILOSOPHICAL BASIS DEFINING THE THERAPEUTIC RELATIONSHIP

Historians of modern medicine have tracked the decline of the centrality of communication over the past seventy years. Shorter notes the ascendancy of molecular- and chemistry-oriented science during the past century and the parallel loss of interest in face-to-face communication. This has resulted in losing focus on the patient as a person. Rather, the patient is viewed in terms of pathological, biomedical, and molecular changes, and this perspective becomes the basis for understanding the patient and for determining what health care will be provided.

I would argue that this shift disregards the value of communication. Furthermore, the medical dialogue has become the fundamental instrument through which the paradigmatic battle for control of the context of the patient's problem is being fought. It is a battle to anchor the patient's problem in either a biomedical or a disease context rather than placing the patient's problem within a broader and more integrated illness context that incorporates the patient's perspective.

The paradigmatic anchor chosen for the medical dialogue determines the nature of the problem, the language that is used to define it, the agenda for the visit, and the therapeutic course to take. The elements of the dialogue define how data is collected, how patient education and counselling is delivered, the nature of the relationship that is built (which is largely in the socio-emotional domain), and how partnership will function (the way in which a mutuality or a collaborative relationship can be established). Figure 1 summarizes the elements of the typical therapeutic visit.

Figure 1
The therapeutic visit

Core elements of the visit	Conceptual groupings of communication elements and functions of the visit

Goals of the visit:
  Physician determined
  Negotiated
  Technical information
  Unclear
	Data gathering
	Patient education and counselling
	Relationship building
	Partnership building

Patient values:
  Assumed
  Explored
  Unexamined	

Physician role:
  Guardian
  Advisor
  Consultant
  Unclear	

Though a relationship of mutuality and collaboration, in which both doctor and patient have high power, has proven the most effective in terms of patient outcomes, it is the one that is most absent in doctor-patient relationships. The power relationships that predominate are paternalism (high doctor power, low patient power), consumerism (high patient power, low doctor power, the doctor being viewed as a "technical consultant"), and default (where neither is in control).

PATIENT CENTREDNESS AND GENDER-LINKED CONVERSATIONAL DIFFERENCES

The ideal interaction, or combination of functional elements of dialogue, has often been described as "patient centred." If you take a functional perspective, the characteristics most often identified in the literature as associated with patient centredness are responsiveness, facilitativeness, informativeness, and participatory communication.

As I define these characteristics and present evidence of their presence in medical interactions, I will also examine how gender affects their patterns. I have chosen to look more closely at gender because it is a potent variable. The literature in the broad field of social psychology is clear on the fact that there are significant gender-linked conversational differences. Highlights from this literature are presented in Figure 2.

Figure 2
Gender-linked conversational differences

In conversations, women in comparison to men

- are more engaging and warm

- use more facial expressions

- smile and gaze more

- touch more

- create less of a distance between themselves,
  and the people they are in conversations with

- use more nonverbal skills

- engage in more self-disclosure

- are less status conscious

In their interactions, women in general like to be close physically, make eye contact, and touch. They are more engaged interpersonally and nod and smile. Women more often disclose things about themselves that are emotionally and psychosocially relevant. They also elicit disclosure from others. Women also tend to affiliate more in exchanges and are less status conscious. They tend to diminish status differentials by affiliative actions, rather than accentuating differences through competitiveness. Women respond to stress by bonding while men often respond with fight or flight.

HOW GENDER AFFECTS THEORETICAL PROTOTYPES AND REFLECTS PRACTICE PATTERNS

Though the above gender conversational differences are well-documented in people's daily lives, are they present in the physician's office? We know that gaining admission to medical school is very difficult, with many more applicants than places available. Medical sociologists have found that successful applicants demonstrate what has been traditionally considered male-linked personality attributes and work habits. These include a single focus, high competitiveness, and the ability to perform regardless of inherent interest. In contrast, women are more often seen as multifocused and affiliative. Even if these attributes do not act to screen women out of the selection process, and it is clear that medical classes in the past five years have been increasingly female, the socialization process of medical school and residency may complete the transformation of females into gender-stripped doctors. Perry Klass's book (1987) about her experiences in medical school at Harvard is telling in this regard. Klass's description of the socialization process in medical school as an extreme ordeal characterized by sleep deprivation and humiliation reveals the dynamics that produce doctors who aspire to practice "macho medicine." Macho medicine considers a "good" doctor to be an aggressive doctor, someone who is definitive, takes control, and makes decisions – someone who is male, or at least male-like.

The hypothesis that follows is that the women who succeed in entering medical school even though they have "gender-linked personality attributes" might lose these during the difficult socialization process. Judy Hall and I have done a number of studies relating physician gender to communication over the years, and we were curious to know if the literature as a whole was consistent with our findings. Our review of the literature produced nineteen communication studies that examined conversational elements related to physician gender. We used only studies that had an empirical record, either an audio- or videotape, and that related some aspect of this communication to physician gender. All studies were of primary care. Many of the gender-linked differences are evident in medical exchanges.

Our analysis revealed that many of the gender-linked differences presented in the sociopsychological literature are present in these studies. I will review some of the main findings concerning gender differences (Roter, Hall, and Aoki 2002; Hall and Roter 2002).

Female physicians are more responsive to patient emotions. They achieve this responsiveness through a greater reliance on emotional statements such as expressions of empathy, self-disclosure, reassurance, and concern. They also use more statements of approval and compliment patients on their efforts (e.g.: "you are looking better"; "you quit smoking, good for you"). They are also more affectively engaged non-verbally, as indicated by head nods, therapeutic touch, smiles, and leaning towards the patient. They more often use a positive tone of voice.

Female physicians are more facilitative. Female physicians conduct longer visits – an average of two and one-half minutes longer than those of male physicians. During the visits, female physicians are less verbally dominant, which means that the patient has more opportunity to speak. They elicit more information from patients in both the biomedical and psychosocial domains; they ask more questions. Interestingly, both male and female patients talk more with a female doctor than with a male one.

Female physicians are more informative. Female physicians give more information to their patients, especially concerning what patients can expect in the psychosocial domain. The psychosocial domain relates to feelings, to emotions, to the daily life of the patient, and to the effects of the patient's disease on the illness experience (how it impacts on relationships and activities with family, friends, workmates, etc.).

Female physicians are more participatory. Female physicians use more partnership statements, which ensures that both speakers are engaged in the process. They check for understanding, seek the patient's opinion, and ask about expectations. Female physicians also seem to be less protective of their status or of their appearance of infallible expertise. A few studies have shown that female physicians will more often consult a reference while the patient is in the room or call in another physician for consultation.

It is relevant to ask how these patterns may translate into outcomes in our health systems. Health systems are changing. In the US, as elsewhere, productivity requirements are pressuring physicians into seeing more patients in shorter time periods. David Mechanic (1996) anticipates that these time pressures will force physicians to abandon socio-emotional aspects of care. Emanuel and Dubler (1995) fear that increased paternalism and limited discussion of patient goals, values, and alternatives may ensue as a result. My thesis is that these time pressures may act to further amplify gender-linked practice differences, as female physicians may find it more difficult to abandon emotional and psychosocial communication than their male colleagues. Female physicians may become the de facto psychosocial experts caring for emotionally distressed and difficult patients. The National Ambulatory Medical Care Survey (NAMCS) reports, which correlate diagnostic categories and physician gender, reveal that women do more psychosocial and mental health diagnosing than men. One might predict that this tendency will be amplified in the future.

This presents significant challenges since female physicians are already at high risk for burnout (as are female nurses). The reasons stem from the strategies they use to make up for longer visits: they work through breaks and lunch and extend their working hours at the end of the day. With visits that are, on average, two and one-half minutes longer, and with an average of thirty patients a day, one might calculate an extra hour of work every day. The time must be found somehow – by skipping breaks or lunch and by working later than male colleagues. Alternatively, one might speculate that time pressures and the stress they create may result in more scheduled revisits, the scheduling of fewer patients per day, or more female physicians opting for part-time employment. Interestingly, Jozien Bensing found in her Dutch study of general practitioners that female doctors working part time have even longer visits than do their full-time counterparts.

CONCLUSION

I will conclude with a series of short statements that capture many years of research on the patient-physician relationship: (1) physician gender matters; (2) health care delivery changes may further amplify these differences; (3) female physicians are at particular risk for burn-out; (4) patient-centred skills are important for all physicians (though I have focused on the differences between male and female physicians, many male doctors use and demonstrate patient centredness, and the overlap is greater than the differences); (5) patient-centred skills can be improved for all doctors through better training and better medical school residency programs.

9

Patient-Practitioner Communication in Conventional and Complementary Medicine Contexts

HEATHER BOON

Every patient knows that the experience of communicating with a health care provider can have a profound effect on how he or she feels. This intuitive knowledge is supported by an increasing amount of research documenting that patient-practitioner communication influences (both positively and negatively) a variety of objective and subjective health outcomes. This chapter begins with an overview of the effects that different physician communication styles may have on patient satisfaction, adherence to treatment protocols, and health outcomes in a conventional medicine context. This is followed by a review of patient-practitioner communication in a complementary medicine context. The perception that complementary practitioners (e.g., naturopathic practitioners, acupuncture practitioners, herbalists) are better communicators than conventional practitioners (e.g., physicians) has been cited as an explanation for why patients seek complementary medicine. The literature supporting this claim is reviewed, and the chapter concludes with a summary of the findings from the first study to directly compare patient-practitioner communication during visits to family physicians and visits to naturopathic practitioners.

PATIENT-PHYSICIAN COMMUNICATION

The Link between Communication and Patient Satisfaction

A review of the literature reveals that physician communication skills are positively correlated with patient reports of satisfaction with care. When patients rate the quality of their communication with the physician highly, they are also more likely to report high levels of satisfaction with the care they receive (Stewart, Brown, Boon, Galajda, Meredith, and Sangster 1999). In fact, the intangible aspects of the patient-practitioner interaction, including communication style, have been reported to be more important in determining patient satisfaction than access or availability issues (Williams and Calnan 1991). In addition, several studies have found a significant link between poor communication and malpractice claims (Beckman, Markakis, Suchman, and Frankel 1994; Hickson, Clayton, Entman, Miller, Githens, Whetten-Goldstein, et al. 1994; Vincent, Young, and Phillips 1994; Hickson, Clayton, Githens, and Sloan 1992; Lester and Smith 1993). It appears that patient satisfaction depends on patients' expectations about their interactions with the physician (Stewart et al. 1999). If what happens in the encounter between patient and physician meshes with the patient's expectations, the patient is more likely to leave the doctor's office satisfied.

Levinson, Roter, Mulloly, Dull, and Frankel (1997) compared the communication styles of primary care physicians who had been the subject of malpractice claims with those who had never experienced a malpractice claim and identified specific communication behaviours that were used by those with "no claims." These included the more frequent use of orientating statements (e.g., explaining to the patient what is about to happen), the appropriate use of humour and laughter, and a greater reliance on facilitating comments (e.g., asking for the patient's opinion, checking for patient understanding). Interestingly, the authors did not find any specific communication behaviours that differentiated *surgeons* with malpractice claims from those who had never been the subject of a malpractice claim. They suggest that factors such as negligence and surgical complications may be more important than communication issues and that this finding may be a result of patients' different expectations of surgeon visits (Levinson et al. 1997).

Communication and Time

There is a widespread belief that good communication requires longer patient-practitioner interactions. Yet the literature on this topic is far from clear. Stewart et al. identify two main themes: (1) that communication style (either positive or negative) is not affected by the length of the interaction and (2) that the length of time available for the interaction does have an effect on the nature of the discussion (Stewart et al. 1999). Several studies have reported that high quality communication is not associated with longer patient visits (Arborelius and Bremberg 1992; Greenfield, Kaplan, Ware, Yano, and Franck 1988; Henbest and Fehrsen 1992). For example, Henbest and Fehrsen (1992) found that more patient-centred interactions took no longer than those that were identified as less patient-centred. However, some studies suggest that patient-practitioner interactions that are more thorough require more time (Hornberger, Thorn, and MaCurdy 1997; Feris 1988; Marvel 1993; Howie, Porter, Heaney, and Hopton 1991; Hull and Hull 1984; Jacobson, Wilkinson, and Owen 1994; Ridsale, Morgan, and Morris 1992; Verby, Holden, and Davis 1979; Westcott 1977). In addition, some topics [e.g., alcohol (Arborelius and Thakker 1995) and stress (Russell and Roter 1993)] and some specific patient groups [e.g., those of low socio-economic status (Bain 1979), teenagers (Hull and Hull 1984), and the elderly (Westcott 1977; Pereles and Russell 1996)] may pose communication difficulties that require longer interactions.

Communication and Adherence

The literature has clearly shown that patient-physician communication is closely correlated with patient adherence to treatment protocols. The following communication factors have been shown to be positively associated with adherence.

Information exchange and patient education. The physician's ability as an educator to ensure that the patient understands and can recall the prescribed treatment protocol has been identified in a number of reviews as a key factor that is closely associated with patient adherence (Kjellgren, Ahlner, and Sakhim 1995; Garrity 1981; Ley 1982; Svarstad 1985). A variety of "communication techniques" that may enhance information exchange and the patient's ability to adhere to treatment protocols have been identified in the literature and include: giving clear, simple directions; repetition; checking for understanding; and the use of communication aids such as diagrams, videos, and written information (Kjellgren et al. 1995; Svarstad 1985; Sanson-Fisher, Campbell, Redman, and Hennrikus 1989; Ley 1985).

Negotiation of mutual expectations. The importance of negotiating treatment goals is identified by a number of studies that report greater adherence when treatment protocols meet both the physician's and the patient's expectations (Garrity 1981; Blackwell 1996; Wilson 1995). In comparison, a mismatch between the expectations of the patient and the physician can result in decreased adherence to the prescribed treatment protocol (Garrity 1981; Blackwell 1996; Golin, Di Matteo, and Gelberg 1996).

Ensuring the patient plays an active role in the interaction. It has been suggested that patients willing to take an active role in making decisions about their treatment protocol are more likely to adhere to the regimen (Garrity 1981; Wilson 1995; Golin et al. 1996). Despite this finding, it is important to note that not all patients desire the same level of involvement in decisions about their care. In addition, desire for participation in clinical decision-making may be time and context dependent (i.e., an individual may desire different levels of decision-making participation for different types of decisions and may desire participation at different times for similar types of decisions) (Golin et al. 1996).

Positive affect from the practitioner. The emotional dimension (sharing, caring, and expressing) has also been associated with increased adherence to treatment protocols (Kjellgren et al. 1995; Garrity 1981). Providing emotional support (Garrity 1981) and empathy (Squier 1990) and working at building a partnership with patients (Roter 1989; Sbarbaro 1990) appear to encourage patients to adhere to treatment protocols.

Communication and patient outcomes. An association between physician communication behaviours and a variety of patient health outcomes has been documented by several literature reviews (Stewart et al. 1999; Stewart 1995). For example, specific elements of the history-taking component of the patient-practitioner interaction (i.e., expressing concern, asking patients for details about their perceptions of the illness experience, asking patients about their feelings, and showing support and empathy) have been shown to decrease patient anxiety, psychological distress, and blood pressure and to increase symptom resolution (Stewart et al. 1999). Specific communication factors during the discussion of the management plan have also been shown to correlate with patient outcomes such as anxiety, pain, increased blood pressure, role and physical limitations, psychological distress, and symptoms resolution (Stewart et al. 1999).

Although this review of the impact of communication on both patient satisfaction and health outcomes is necessarily brief, it clearly demonstrates that physician communication style and skill has a great influence on the patient's perception of both the encounter itself and the illness experience. It has been argued that poor physician communication is one factor that has led to the increasing use of complementary medicine.

COMPLEMENTARY MEDICINE

Complementary medicine – also known as alternative medicine or complementary/alternative medicine (CAM) – can be defined as "healing resources that encompass all health systems, modalities, and practices and their accompanying theories and beliefs, other than those intrinsic to the politically dominant health system of a particular society or culture in a given historical period. CAM includes all such practices and ideas self-defined by their users as preventing or treating illness or promoting health and well-being" (National Institutes of Health [US] Panel of Definition and Description 1997). Examples of complementary medicine include: alternative medical systems such as traditional Chinese medicine and naturopathic medicine; mind-body interventions such as meditation; biological-based therapies such as herbs and supplements; manipulative and body-based therapies such as chiropractic and massage; and energy therapies such as therapeutic touch and Reiki. An estimated 42–50 per cent of Canadians are reported to use some form of complementary medicine (Ramsay, Walker, and Alexander 1999; CTV/Angus Reid Group 1997), and the use of these products and therapies by North Americans appears to be growing (Eisenberg, Davis, Ettener, et al. 1998).

Reasons Patients Seek Complementary Medicine

It has been suggested that the increasing popularity of complementary medicine is a product of consumer dissatisfaction with the present health care system (Gray, Greenberg, Fitch, Parry, Douglas, and Labrecque 1997; Alster 1989; British Medical Association 1986; Berliner and Salmon 1980; Wiesner 1989; van Dam 1986). One hypothesis is that the special relationship that develops between complementary medicine practitioners and their patients is key to understanding why patients seek this type of care (Sellerberg 1991). Patient relationships with complementary medicine practitioners are thought to differ from those that develop between patients and physicians in three key ways. First, complementary medicine practitioners spend more time with each patient (thirty to sixty minutes per visit in many cases) (Goldstein, Sutherland, Jaffe, and Wilson 1988; Boon 1998a). Second, complementary practitioners are thought to have more equal, open, and reciprocal relationships with their patients (Goldstein et al. 1988; Sharma 1994). Finally, it is hypothesized that complementary practitioners form stronger psychosocial bonds with patients (Goldstein et al. 1988; Hewer 1983) than physicians. There is some direct evidence to support the claim that complementary practitioners spend more time with patients. However, there is virtually no information about whether relationships with complementary practitioners are in fact less hierarchical or whether the type of bond that forms between complementary practitioners and their patients differs in any significant way from the bonds physicians develop with their patients. Additional research is needed before any conclusions can be drawn about whether communication between complementary practitioners and their patients plays a role in explaining why patients seek their care.

PILOT STUDY COMPARING VISITS
TO FAMILY PHYSICIANS (FPS)
AND NATUROPATHIC PRACTITIONERS (NPS)

We conducted a pilot study to compare the interactions of patients with naturopathic practitioners (NPs) and with family physicians (FPs). NPs can be described as general practitioners in complementary medicine contexts. They are trained in a variety of treatment modalities – including botanical medicine, clinical nutrition, homeopathic medicine, oriental medicine and acupuncture, and naturopathic manipulation – and are currently regulated in four Canadian provinces: British Columbia, Saskatchewan, Manitoba, and Ontario. FPs are primary care physicians who have completed a two-year residency program in family medicine and who are licensed by provincial colleges of family physicians according to standards maintained by the Canadian College of Family Physicians.

A convenience sample of ten practitioners (five NPs and five FPs) from southern Ontario (Canada) agreed to participate in this study. NPs and FPs were matched according to: gender, number of years in practice, and practice location. Each practitioner was asked to enrol the first three consecutive patients (starting on a day specified by the investigator) presenting with "new complaints" who agreed to participate. All patient-practitioner interactions were audio-taped and transcribed verbatim. Additional data were collected by using both questionnaires that included a patient-centredness scale and follow-up qualitative interviews with patients. A total of seventeen patients (twelve of whom visited NPs and fifteen of whom visited FPs) were enrolled in this pilot study.

Patient-Centredness

The patient-centred model used in this study was developed by Levenstein (1984) and researchers at the University of Western Ontario (Levenstein, McCracken, McWhinney, Stewart, and Brown 1986; McCracken, Stewart, Brown, and McWhinney 1983). It is made up of six interconnecting components. The first three components encompass the communication process between the patient and doctor: (1) exploring the disease and illness experience (patient feelings, ideas, perceptions of effect on function and expectations); (2) understanding the whole person; and (3) finding common ground between the patient and the practitioner. The second set of three components focuses on the context in which the patient and the practitioner interact: (4) incorporation of prevention and health promotion; (5) enhancing the patient-practitioner relationship; and (6) being realistic (using available resources, energy, and time).

There was no significant difference between the FP patients' and the NP patients' overall scores on the nine-item patient centredness score. Further analysis did not find any significant difference on any of the three sub-scales: perception that the illness was fully explored, perception that common ground was found, and perception that the patient was treated as a whole (see Table 1).

Communication Issues

During qualitative interviews conducted in the week following their visits to the study practitioner, patients were asked to identify the "best" characteristic or part of their interaction with the study practitioner. Three themes were identified by both FP and NP patients: the importance of having a practitioner who "really listened," being encouraged (and feeling comfortable enough) to ask questions, and feeling that the practitioner "really cared" about them as individuals. NP patients identified one additional theme: a practitioner that was interested in finding out about their symptoms or concerns in the context of their whole life story.

The importance of a practitioner who "really listened" was an important theme raised by both the FP patients and the NP patients. Almost all the patients in the study identified their practitioners as true listeners: "He spent the time and really listened to everything I had to say. He took all my suggestions seriously... I was being listened to as a human being. I wasn't a number." This theme was clearly identified by the patients as inextricably linked to their satisfaction with the practitioner they were visiting. Many told stories of other practitioners "who didn't listen" and identified this as a major reason for switching practitioners. Both NP and FP patients felt very strongly that listening skills were an important characteristic of a "good" practitioner.

A second related theme was the ability of the practitioner to create an atmosphere that encouraged the patient to ask questions. Both FP and NP patients contrasted their present practitioners with "bad practitioners" they had visited previously who had made them feel "stupid for asking questions." Both groups of patients identified "good" practitioners as those who appeared eager to answer patient questions and

Table 1
Patients' and physicians' perceptions of patient-centredness

Item	Mean score (lower scores indicate more positive response)		
	NP patients (n = 12)	FP patients (n = 15)	P value (T-test)
Perception that illness was explored (composite score) To what extent was your main problem discussed today? To what extent did the doctor listen to what you had to say? How well do you think your practitioner understood you today?	1.56	1.31	0.233
Perception that common ground was found (composite score) How satisfied were you with the discussion of your patient's problem? To what extent did you explain the problem to your patient? To what extent did you and the patient discuss you respective roles? To what extent did you explain treatment? To what extent did you explore how manageable this (treatment) would be for the patient?	2.08	1.64	0.885
Perception of treatment as a whole person To what extent did you discuss personal or family issues that might affect your patient's health?	2.56	1.81	0.662
Overall perception of patient-centredness	1.95	1.56	0.139

who provided detailed explanations when necessary. Patients in both groups also described practitioners who "really cared about their patients" as "good" practioners. Patients had great difficulty articulating what their practitioners actually did or said to make them feel cared for, but it was clearly identified as a desirable characteristic of both FPs and NPs.

One final theme came up in discussion with NP patients only: the provision of "holistic care." NP patients identified "good" practitioners as those who were interested in finding out about patients' symptoms or concerns in the context of their whole life stories: "He looks at me as a whole human being, not [as] just a liver patient or a heart patient or whatever." This idea of "holistic care" is particularly important because some of the patients who sought care from NPs in our study were not ill by biomedical standards: they didn't have a diagnosed disease, and they didn't suffer from any serious troubles or symptoms. Nonetheless, they wanted advice about becoming "healthier."

Time

Time – both in terms of the amount of time practitioners spend with patients and with respect to feelings of having "enough" time – was a very important theme to these patients. Visits to NPs lasted on average 54.0 minutes (range 30.4 to 92.9 minutes), which was significantly longer than the average FP visit (16.5 minutes, range 8.3 to 26.1 minutes). NP patients explained that having more time meant that the relationship could develop more quickly and allowed patients to explain their problems and concerns in detail: "I spent two and a half hours with him [the naturopath] last Thursday. I've had the same physician for twenty years now, and I told the naturopath more last Thursday than I've told my doctor in twenty years."

Taking all the time necessary was a key theme. Although NPs spent more time with their patients, many of the FPs' patients felt their practitioners had taken all the time necessary to deal with all of their issues. Patients said that if an issue could not be concluded in one encounter, the physician made sure to book another visit. In other cases, the physician said s/he would look up some information and get back to the patient. So, from these patients' point of view, it was not so much the time per se spent during the visit that was important, but rather the impression that there was enough time to deal with all the issues. In some cases, this could be done in a short time span.

CONCLUSION

Communication issues clearly have a significant impact on patient-practitioner relationships. Good practitioner communication skills are generally associated with higher levels of patient satisfaction, patient adherence to treatments, and patient health outcomes. Although it has been argued that patients seek the care of complementary/alternative medicine practitioners because they develop stronger psychological bonds in less hierarchical relationships with these practitioners in comparison to their relationships with conventional practitioners, this claim is not currently supported by empirical evidence. Our pilot study results suggest that patients do not perceive any difference in the patient-centredness of their interactions with NPs and FPs. In addition, NP and FP patients identified very similar characteristics of "good" practitioners, describing them as those who listen to patients, encourage questions, and make patients feel cared for. There is some evidence that "good" communication does not necessarily require more time; however, it is clear that spending more time with patients has implications for the development of relationships. In this discussion, time is a key factor that requires further investigation.

10

An Interpersonal Social Support Approach to Understanding the Patient-Practitioner Relationship

KRISTA K. TROBST

Technological advances and medical breakthroughs have given the physician the ability to diagnose and treat that would have been considered science fiction only years ago. Yet, in spite of these great discoveries – or in part because of them – all is not well with modern medicine. For all the growth we have witnessed on the technical side of medicine, the interpersonal side, involving the human element of care, has not kept pace.

Bernard and Krupat 1994, 115

The practice of medicine has probably always been concerned with enhancing the diagnosis and treatment of what ails us. However, more interpersonal considerations of "quality of care" seem to be primarily a product of the last few decades – at least from a research, rather than from a merely intuitive, standpoint. In fact, relatively recent times have been witness to a blossoming of research examining the inter-personal quality of patient-practitioner[1] (or patient-physician, or patient-provider) relationships, including considerations not only of what patients like in their practitioners, but also of how patients' health might benefit from good relationships with their practitioners. Perhaps not surprisingly, it seems that it *does* matter whether or not we like our health care practitioners. In general, we evaluate the care we receive from our practitioners along many of the same lines as we do the social support we receive from our friends, spouses, and family

---

1 The term "patient-practitioner" will be used here to encompass not only patient-physician relationships, but also relationships with other health care practitioners, including nurses, physiotherapists, chiropractors, naturopaths, etc., in keeping with the more differentiated aspects of health care provision that comprise our most modern approach to "medicine."

members; we benefit more from their actions when we feel cared for. With respect to our health care practitioners, the feeling of being cared for affects both our satisfaction with care and our willingness to follow through with treatment recommendations.

This chapter, in addition to outlining some of what we have learned about patient-practitioner relationships, will focus on a reconceptualization of health care services as something provided within an interpersonal social support context. Social support research began in earnest at approximately the same time as patient-practitioner research, but the findings generated in each field have been utilized independently of each other. I believe, however, that through the application of social support research we can increase the sophistication of our theoretical and measurement approaches to understanding patient-practitioner relationships. Doing so, however, requires that we begin with the premise that when practitioners interact with patients they are, in any of several ways, providing social support, not just technical services. We will return to this issue later in the chapter, but first I will present a brief summary of research examining the patient-practitioner relationship.

PATIENT-PRACTITIONER
RELATIONSHIP RESEARCH

For many years, researchers have investigated the relationships between patients and their health care practitioners, be they physicians, nurses, dentists, or technicians, among many other possible categories. Of particular concern has been: (1) the sorts of things that make us satisfied or dissatisfied with the care we receive and (2) what effect our level of satisfaction has on our health care behaviours. For example, are we prone to liking practitioners who listen, express concern, or seem confident? Are we more likely to follow advice in adopting that "oh so difficult" exercise program, or low fat diet, or arduous medical regimen if we like and are satisfied with the practitioner who prescribed it?

Most of us have had both positive and negative experiences in our dealings with health care providers, but most of us seldom think about the specifics of what impressed or alienated us, or about what effect these feelings might have had on our willingness to follow through with treatment recommendations. Research on patient-practitioner relationships has, however, begun to establish what sorts of things we do and don't want in a health care provider.

It would certainly seem that the most important characteristic in a health care provider would be competence because, after all, our health and well-being are at stake! Clearly, we do want competent health care (Thom and Campbell 1997), but competence does not seem to be the primary criteria by which we evaluate our care (Ben-Sira 1976, 1980; Ware, Davies-Avery, and Stewart 1978b). Research has demonstrated that people often judge the adequacy of their care by criteria that are irrelevant to its technical quality (Gough 1967), and warm providers are often judged to be more competent than providers who are not as warm (Buller and Buller 1987; Di Matteo, Linn, Chang, and Cope 1985). This is perhaps less surprising when you consider that most of us don't have enough medical knowledge to judge technical competence, except in the more extreme cases, and then probably mostly when a lack of competence is involved. So, instead, it seems we pay more attention to the manner in which care is delivered – i.e., to "the interpersonal aspects of health care."

What do we want in a physician or other health care provider? Research to date has shown that we want a warm, confident, and friendly provider (Buller and Buller 1987; Di Matteo, Linn, Chang, and Cope 1985; Roberts and Aruguete 2000) who is receptive (Burgoon et al. 1987), who gives us feedback (Delbanco et al. 2001), who provides emotional support (Marvel, Doherty, and Weiner 1998), and who is relatively egalitarian, including us in decision making (Thom and Campbell 1997). When presented with such a provider, we are likely to be satisfied with our health care. In fact, it appears that the practice of "doctor shopping" is primarily based not on a consideration of the competence of the practitioner, but on a desire to find a physician whose interpersonal behaviour fulfils our needs for caring and concern (Di Matteo, Prince, and Taranta 1979; Kasteler, Kane, Olsen, and Thetford 1976; Safran, Montgomery, Chang, Murphy, and Rogers 2001). But, as mentioned earlier, we are also likely to judge less caring practitioners as less competent, although in reality interpersonal skills and medical competence are not related (Gough 1967); we are about as likely to receive top quality, highly competent care from the aloof physician as we are from the nurturing one.

By extension, then, what we don't want in a health care practitioner becomes fairly obvious. Following are some patient complaints regarding health care providers.

Lack of competence or skill. When we visit health care practitioners we clearly want them to diagnose us appropriately and to provide treatment that will remedy the problem or at least alleviate any discomfort we may be experiencing. We are therefore more likely to be satisfied with practitioners who succeed in doing so and are likely to be dissatisfied with those who don't. This may be particularly the case when dealing with an acute symptom like pain from which we want to, and expect to, find relief at the hands of our practitioners (Sherwood, Adams-McNeill, Starck, Nieto, and Thompson 2000).

Expressing uncertainty about the nature of the condition. Perhaps obviously, having a health care practitioner express bafflement about one's condition can be highly disconcerting, although there are many circumstances in which such uncertainty would be justified and would not at all reflect a lack of knowledge or competence on the part of the provider. Nonetheless, overall we expect our practitioners to be able to definitively diagnose and treat our conditions and we respond poorly to displays of incertitude (Johnson, Levenkron, Suchman, and Manchester 1988).

Dominance/decision-making. Individuals will likely differ in the extent to which they want to be involved in medical decision-making (Krantz, Baum, and Wideman 1980) and, by extension, in the degree to which they would prefer a dominant or more egalitarian physician. For example, elderly patients often appear to prefer having their practitioners make the medical decisions for them (Woodward and Wallston 1987). In general, however, it appears that patients are more satisfied with practitioners who are less dominant and controlling (Burgoon et al. 1987; Cecil 1998).

Not listening. We don't like to be interrupted or prevented from finishing our explanations of what symptoms we are experiencing, and research suggests that these feelings are well-warranted. One study, for example, monitored the interactions between over seventy physicians and their patients and found that, on average, a patient is interrupted after eighteen seconds of speech (Beckman and Frankel 1984). In addition to being annoying and dismissive, a great deal of potentially valuable information may be lost through such exchanges (Roter and Hall 1987).

Use of jargon (technical language). Many health care providers are prone to using technical language in their interactions with their patients (Di Matteo and Di Nicola 1982; McKinlay 1975; Musialowski 1988; Ventres and Gordon 1990), and a number of reasons have been suggested for this, ranging from the benign to the malignant. For example, practitioners may use jargon to keep the patient from asking too many questions, to hide uncertainty about the patient's condition, or to impress the patient and maintain a status differential (Waitzkin 1985). The more benign, and perhaps more reasonable, explanations include the argument that the use of jargon is simply an automatic behaviour, carried over from physicians' educational experiences, and that it results from a simple lack of perspective-taking ability with respect to deciphering what patients likely can and cannot understand. This is in keeping with other research suggesting that physicians' behaviours may be hampered by less than ideal (although no less than normal) perspective-taking abilities; that is, research has found that there is little relation between a patient's rating of satisfaction and the physician's rating of that patient's satisfaction (Hall, Stein, Roter, and Rieser 1999).

Baby talk. At the opposite extreme of jargon, health care providers sometimes engage in "baby talk" or overly simplistic language, which is often perceived as condescension (Toynbee 1977). Perhaps more importantly, however, in its overly simplistic form, such language also leads to the provision of little useful data and to the omission of much information from which patients might truly benefit.

Depersonalization of the patient. Patients respond poorly to depersonalized health care (Deckard, Meterko, and Field 1994; Kaufman 1970). From the practitioner's perspective, objectifying the patient may allow the provider to concentrate on the condition rather than on the person, and it provides emotional protection for the practitioner. However, from the patient's perspective, depersonalization often comes across as cold and uncaring.

Taken together, research has shown that providers who engage in behaviours of these sorts are judged by patients to be not only unfriendly, but also incompetent, however unwarranted the latter judgment might be. And, although many health care providers would be loathe to see a portion of their job as involving a need to engage in "popularity contests," there are bona fide reasons for satisfying one's patients.

THE PATIENT-PRACTITIONER RELATIONSHIP IN PATIENT COMPLIANCE

Research has shown that patients who are dissatisfied with their physicians are less likely to continue to use health care services in the future (Ross and Duff 1982), are more likely to change physicians (Di Matteo et al. 1979; Kasteler et al. 1976), are less likely to comply with treatment recommendations (Sherbourne, Hays, Ordway, Di Matteo, and Kravitz 1992), and are more likely to file complaints, including malpractice suits (Frankel 1995; Hayes-Bautista 1976; Ware, Davies-Avery,

and Stewart 1978b). A particular focus in research endeavours has
been the effect that such dissatisfaction has on the critical issue of
patient compliance with treatment recommendations.

Establishing estimates of compliance or adherence – that is, of the
degree to which individuals follow their prescribed treatment regimens
– has proven very difficult due to differences in types of regimens (from
taking medication to undergoing surgery or chemotherapy, to exercis-
ing or eating a low fat diet) and the multiple ways in which we can
fail to follow advice. For example, patients can take too much or too
little medication or take doses at the wrong times (Di Matteo 1995),
or partially but not entirely follow exercise or diet recommendations.
Although estimates of compliance vary widely, 40 per cent noncompliance, or 60 per cent compliance, might serve as an overall estimate
(Di Matteo and Lepper 1998). More germane here, however, are the
findings regarding the interpersonal aspects of care and their relation
to compliance.

Taken together, it appears that warmth begets compliance and that
apparent disinterest or impatience begets noncompliance (Sherbourne
et al. 1992; Garrity 1981; Ley 1982). Also, with respect to malpractice
litigation, the most obvious sign of patient discontent, such suits are
much more likely to be waged against physicians who, regardless of
overall competence, are fearful, insecure, or derogatory (Blum 1957,
1960) and who have shorter visits with their patients (Levinson, Roter,
Mullooly, Dull, and Frankel 1997).

Clearly, we have learned a great deal about patient-practitioner relationships from the research that has been conducted to date. On the
more practical side, this kind of research has led to the very useful
application of this knowledge in teaching practitioners how to better
communicate with their patients (e.g., Harvard Medical School's New
Pathways program; Tosteson, Adelstein, and Carver 1994). Nonetheless, there are some problems within this area of research. In particular,
many of the measures that are currently used to assess constructs such
as the nature of the patient-practitioner interaction, or patient satisfaction with practitioners, lack sophistication in that they are often
poorly constructed and lack reliability and/or validity. Also, there
appear to be few agreed-upon measures, and researchers therefore
often construct a measure for their own use and employ different
measures from one study to the next, thereby not allowing for a
comparison of the various measures and a determination of which ones
are better than the rest. For example, between 1986 and 1996, one
study (Boon and Stewart 1998b) examined instruments developed to
assess patient-provider interactions or satisfaction levels. This study
found forty-four different measures, thirty-six of which were either

used in only one study or not supported by sufficient information about the qualities of the test to evaluate its desirability; hence virtually no information was available for choosing the best or better measures.

I will now turn my attention to what I think may be a suitable alternative approach to examining patient-practitioner relationships – one that makes use of an interpersonal theory and measurement model of social support.

AN INTERPERSONAL CONCEPTUALIZATION OF SOCIAL SUPPORT

Social support research began in earnest with a highly influential paper by the epidemiologist Sidney Cobb in 1976 in which he discussed the importance of social support for mediating health outcomes. A flurry of research followed that continued to demonstrate that social support plays an important role in predicting the severity of physiological and psychological symptoms (Schwarzer and Leppin 1989). Also, although we tend to think of social support as emanating from our friends and families, our health care providers are also in a social support role; indeed, it appears that Dr Cobb also had health care practitioners in mind when he formulated his conceptualization of social support.

Cobb defined social support as "information leading the subject to believe that he is cared for and loved, esteemed, and a member of a network of mutual obligations" (1976, 300). He went on to say, by way of example, "that a competently staffed hospital [that] is available in case of need is socially supportive." His emphasis, however, was not on the activities or technical services performed in such a setting, but on the manner in which they are performed.

The present meaning of social support does not include the activities of the hospital in repairing a broken leg. Those activities are material services and are not of themselves information of any of the major classes mentioned above. This does not mean that the *deferential manner* of the intern may not provide esteem support or that the *tender care* of the nurses may not communicate emotional support. It is only to say that the services do not in themselves constitute such support. (301, emphases added)

Cobb's emphasis in defining support was on those actions that convey a sense of caring and esteem, suggesting two dimensions that are highly similar to the two axes of a structural model of interpersonal behaviour called the Interpersonal Circumplex Model or ICM (Leary 1957; Wiggins 1979). Within this model, the axes can be interpreted at different levels of abstraction (see Figure 1) ranging from the metatheoretical

Figure 1
Levels of interpretation of circumplex axes

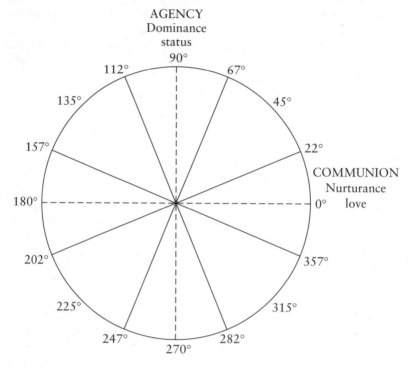

AGENCY
Dominance
status

constructs of agency and communion to dominance and nurturance, and at an even lower level to status and love (Trobst 1999).

Using this model as a guide, I set out several years ago to construct a circumplex measure of social support that has come to be called the Support Actions Scale Circumplex (SAS-C) (Trobst 1999, 2000; Wiggins and Trobst 1997b). This seemed a worthwhile endeavour not only because interpersonal theory and measurement has much to recommend it (Kiesler 1996; Wiggins and Trobst 1997a), but also because social support research was plagued by many of the same problems that occur in patient-practitioner relationship research. For example, there was little agreement among researchers regarding what form a social support measure should take; thus various measures proliferated, some of which were not well developed or properly validated and many of which were used in only one or a handful of studies. By extension, there was no theory or model to guide the development of these measures or to dictate either what components should be included or how to refer to those components. For example, should we refer to expressions of caring as emotional support, as love, as relatedness, or as belonging? Similarly, should we refer to respectful actions as esteem support, as affirmation, or as social reinforcement? Nonetheless, what was clear was that many researchers in the area made reference to forms of support reminiscent of the ICM themes of providing love and status to others. Table 1 lists some of the investigators who discuss these forms of love and status support under various guises.

However, further description of the model would seem to be in order if we are to determine how a model that contains love and status as its axes might serve to improve our conceptualization and measurement of social support and/or patient-practitioner relationships. Figure 2 illustrates the basic ICM structure, with directive (or status) behaviours at the top and avoidant (or submissive) behaviours at the bottom, and with nurturant (or love) behaviours on the right and critical (or cold) behaviours on the left. The lines dividing the circle are essentially arbitrarily placed but conform to what has become the standard convention in ICM models – they divide the circle into eight sectors referred to as octants. The degree symbols indicate the boundaries of these sectors and their midpoints, and the letter designations

Table 1
Love and status in the social support literature

Author	Care (i.e., love)	Esteem (i.e., status)
Caplan 1974	Emotional mastery	Feedback
Weiss 1974	Attachment	Reassurance of worth
Cobb 1976	Love	Esteem
Tolsdorf 1976	Intangible	Feedback
Gottlieb 1978	Concern	Respect
Hirsch 1980	Emotional support	Social reinforcement
Barrera, Sandler, and Ramsay 1981	Intimate interaction	Feedback
House 1981	Emotional support	Appraisal support
Kahn and Antonucci 1981	Affect	Affirmation
Cohen and Hoberman 1983	Belonging	Self-esteem
Schumaker and Brownell 1984	Affiliative needs	Self-esteem enhancement
Cutrona 1986	Emotional support	Esteem support
Hobfoll 1988	Love	Esteem
Vaux 1988	Love and affection	Esteem and identity
Sarason, Sarason, and Pierce 1990	Love	Esteem
Ryan and Solky 1996	Relatedness	Autonomy

Source: Copyright 2000 Sage Publications Inc. Reprinted, with permission of the publisher, from K.K. Trobst, "An interpersonal conceptualization and quantification of social support transactions," *Personality and Social Psychology Bulletin* 26 (2000): 972.

Figure 2
The Support Actions Scale Circumplex (SAS-C)

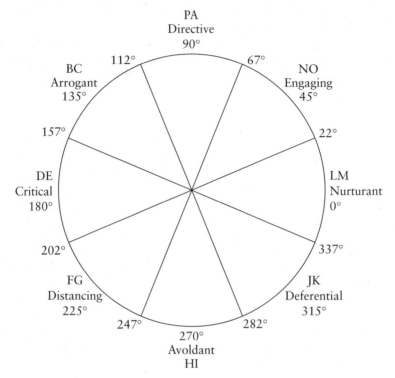

of PA, BC, DE, etc. designate the location of the sector. These labels stem from the originators of the circumplex (Freedman, Leary, Ossario, and Coffey 1951), who initially had devised sixteen sectors within the circle. It was subsequently decided that the use of eight sectors might be more workable and easier to understand. Labelling therefore now includes a two-letter designation for each octant, beginning with PA at the top of the circle and moving in a counter-clockwise direction.]

The labels given to each octant (Directive, Arrogant, etc.) vary from one ICM measure to another depending on the interpersonal domain under investigation and the content of the items included. For example, whereas the premier circumplex measure of normal interpersonal traits (Interpersonal Adjective Scales) (Wiggins 1995) labels the PA octant "Assured-Dominant," the leading circumplex measure of problems in interpersonal behaviour (Inventory of Interpersonal Problems Circumplex) (Horowitz, Alden, Wiggins, and Pincus 2000) labels the PA octant

"Domineering," and the SAS-C labels the PA octant "Directive." In all instances, PA denotes dominant behaviours, but the most appropriate summary label for expressing the nature of those behaviours varies across content areas.

With respect to the SAS-C (see Figure 2), the PA (Directive) sector includes dominant social support behaviours in relatively pure form (i.e., they are neither particularly warm nor cold), such as "giving advice." As we move in a counterclockwise direction to BC (Arrogant), we are moving towards the cold dimension; thus these behaviours are a blend of dominance and coldness and include items such as "persuade them to change their behaviour." DE (Critical) behaviours are relatively cold, although not particularly dominant nor submissive, and include items such as "tell them they have to learn to live with it." FG (Distancing) behaviours move towards the submissive pole and are a blend of submissive and cold behaviours (e.g., "try to keep them from leaning on me too much"). HI (Avoidant) behaviours are a relatively pure form of submission and include items such as "avoid giving any advice." JK (Deferential) behaviours involve both warmth and submission (e.g., "remain non-judgmental"). LM (Nurturant) behaviours are nurturant and warm and include items such as "be careful not to pressure them." And NO (Engaging) behaviours are both warm and dominant (e.g., "check up on them frequently").

It should be noted at this point, however, that the SAS-C was not explicitly developed for the assessment of patient-practitioner relationships; rather it was designed to capture the support behaviours of close others (e.g., friends or family members). As such, some of the item content of the SAS-C is particular to close relationships and would not translate well or be relevant to the assessment of patient-practitioner relationships (e.g., an item from the NO scale such as "try to involve them in social activities"). Additional research is therefore needed to particularize the SAS-C for the assessment of patient-practitioner relationships, although the SAS-C *model* (if not its *measurement*) might serve to elucidate the nature of the domain under consideration in a more multifaceted (and theory-driven and psychometrically precise) manner than has previously been achieved.

One of the primary features of the SAS-C that serves to differentiate it from other models and measures of social support (or patient-practitioner) behaviours is that it is not only multifaceted, but also bipolar in nature. As a result, it surveys not only the prototypically warm and accepting actions one could provide in a support situation, but also several forms of more challenging, dismissive, or avoidant actions. People behave in various ways when presented with the need to provide support, and fortunately we usually fill our support roles reasonably well, but sometimes we don't handle the situation effectively, becoming aloof, hostile, overly dominant, or overly submissive. This model allows both the good and the bad of support exchanges to be captured.

There are clearly many other models and measures of social support behaviour, but the present model seems to have much to recommend it. In addition to its theoretical underpinnings and psychometric precision, the SAS-C appears to capture a much broader array of social support behaviour than is typically assessed with other commonly employed measures. This issue was examined by asking respondents to complete the SAS-C and several other commonly used measures of support. The findings indicated (see Figure 3) that the majority of the existing social support scales fall within or close to the border of the SAS-C Engaging (NO) octant. Actions located within this octant are associated with the granting of both love and status to others (that is, with both emotional and esteem support) and are thus clearly consistent with common notions of supportive behaviour. However, despite attempts to distinguish different classes of resources that might be provided in a support context, like financial and practical assistance, all of these behaviours were provided disproportionately by individuals adopting an Engaging (NO) support style. What is most important for the present purposes, however, is that it appears that the SAS-C delineates a variety of behaviours that occur in support contexts that have not been systematically captured by existing inventories. As a result, the SAS-C appears to be a promising inventory, but that promise can only be established through future research.

With respect to patient-practitioner relationship research, there is even more work to be done, the first step of which is to establish the SAS-C model and measure as suitable for application within that domain. The model itself would seem to be directly applicable; practitioner behaviour varies in terms of dominance and nurturance along the same lines as all other forms of interpersonal behaviour. And the application of this theoretically rich perspective would certainly advance research in this area. The ICM measurement aspect is also highly promising, although future research will need to alter and fine-tune the instrument for use in this particular context.

Nonetheless, within the present context, I provide Figure 4 as an illustration of the potential of this model for elucidating patient-practitioner relationships. We have discussed the good and the bad of practitioner behaviour or, expressed another way, what we do and don't like in our health care practitioners. Taking what we know so far in this area, I have taken the liberty of tentatively mapping some of those practitioner behaviours onto the SAS-C as a means of illustration and hypothesis generation.

Figure 3
Projections of other social support measures onto the SAS-C

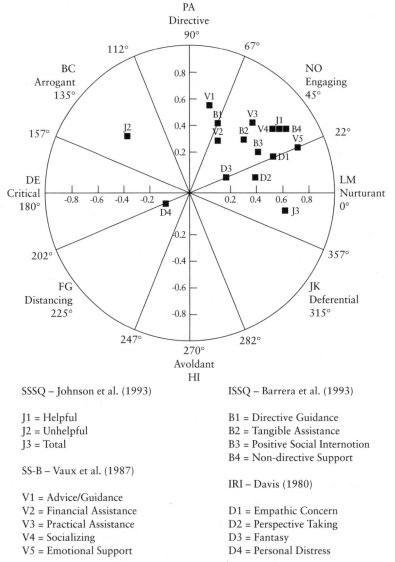

SSSQ – Johnson et al. (1993)

J1 = Helpful
J2 = Unhelpful
J3 = Total

SS-B – Vaux et al. (1987)

V1 = Advice/Guidance
V2 = Financial Assistance
V3 = Practical Assistance
V4 = Socializing
V5 = Emotional Support

ISSQ – Barrera et al. (1993)

B1 = Directive Guidance
B2 = Tangible Assistance
B3 = Positive Social Internotion
B4 = Non-directive Support

IRI – Davis (1980)

D1 = Empathic Concern
D2 = Perspective Taking
D3 = Fantasy
D4 = Personal Distress

Source: Copyright 2000 Sage Publications Inc. Reprinted, with permission of the publisher, from K.K. Trobst, "An interpersonal conceptualization and quantification of social support transactions," *Personality and Social Psychology Bulletin* 26 (2000): 980.

Figure 4
Conceptualizing practitioner behaviours within the sas-c framework

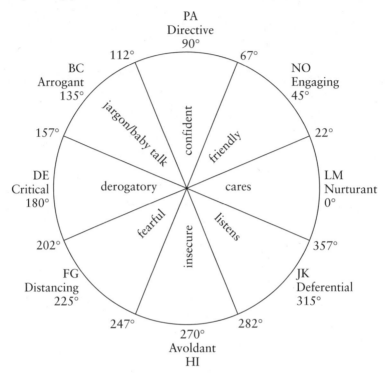

Beginning with Directive (PA) at the top of the circle, we can surmise that confidence in a practitioner is likely to be a desirable characteristic that serves to enhance our satisfaction with care, although if the practitioner demonstrates confidence in such a way as to become overly controlling or dominant, this behaviour may undermine our satisfaction. Such a movement towards controlling behaviour, however, is more likely to be captured within the adjacent (counterclockwise) Arrogant (BC) octant, and this form of behaviour is also likely to be associated with the use of technical language (jargon) and/or baby talk that serve to reaffirm the superior status of the practitioner but also serve to annoy the patient and diminish the quality of the relationship. Critical (DE) behaviours are likely to involve a lack of sympathy for the patient's plight and a tendency to blame and criticize the patient – behaviours that are likely to have a significant negative effect on patient satisfaction. Distancing (FG) actions would likely characterize the fearful practitioner and might include attempts to avoid discussion of emotions and to discourage the patient from becoming reliant upon the practitioner; these behaviours are also likely to be associated with patient dissatisfaction.

Avoidant (HI) behaviours are submissive and would likely characterize the insecure practitioner; they include a lack of willingness to give advice or make recommendations. Although many patients are likely to be averse to controlling behaviours, patients are also likely to be dissatisfied with a practitioner who is reluctant to suggest and guide behaviours and treatments. Many patients (probably particularly self-assured and/or knowledgeable ones) are, however, likely to be relatively satisfied with a practitioner who engages in Deferential (JK) behaviours because, although somewhat submissive in quality, such actions include listening and being non-argumentative and non-judgmental. Among the most desirable of practitioner behaviours, however, are likely Nurturant (LM) actions, which include listening, being patient, and providing emotional support. Similarly, Engaging (NO) actions are likely to be significantly associated with patient satisfaction due to the enthusiasm, concern, and protective qualities they engender.

The foregoing should, however, be treated only as a source for hypothesis generation; empirical research is clearly needed to establish the veridicality of these suppositions. Nonetheless, it is hoped that this discussion has also served to highlight the potential benefit of this kind of multifaceted approach to understanding the very human, interpersonal qualities of patient-practitioner interactions.

Dynamic Conceptions of Dimensions in the Interpersonal Domain

D.S. MOSKOWITZ

Many of the methodologies, conceptual frameworks, and general issues raised in psychology can be applied to the study of health care providers and health care receivers. I will offer some insights into how both our feelings and our behaviours fluctuate, the factors that impact on them, and how knowing about these dynamics and employing them can be useful in the health care field.

AFFECT AND BEHAVIOUR FLUCTUATE

Both how we feel and how we behave fluctuate. How we feel can change rapidly or slowly in the course of minutes, or hours, or days. Behaviour also fluctuates. We tend to speak of others as being either warm and friendly or cold and quarrelsome when in fact most people are friendly at some times and quarrelsome at other times. It is often possible to know how a person feels by how that person is behaving. This is because affect and behaviour often fluctuate together. The extent to which behaviour and affect co-fluctuate is a function of at least two characteristics of the interaction: (1) the qualities of the situation itself (for example, the role relationship between people) and (2) the characteristics that the individual brings into the interaction.

To monitor these fluctuations, I work with the Interpersonal Circumplex Model. A simplified version of this model is presented below in Figure 1.

As indicated in the model, behaviours we adopt when interacting with others vary along two dimensions: (1) the agentic dimension, which refers to the extent or balance of dominant and submissive

Figure 1
Interpersonal Circumplex Model

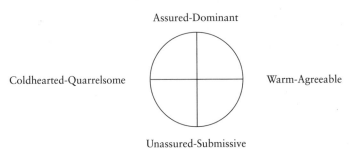

Assured-Dominant

Coldhearted-Quarrelsome

Warm-Agreeable

Unassured-Submissive

behaviours, and (2) the communal dimension, which refers to the extent or balance of agreeable and quarrelsome behaviours. These dimensions are independent of each other. Thus we can engage in dominant behaviour either in an agreeable fashion or in a quarrelsome fashion. We can also engage in submissive behaviour while being either agreeable or quarrelsome (Moskowitz 1994a; Wiggins 1991).

Another way to view these dimensions is to consider what the individual is seeking when engaging in interactions. The person's objective may involve status and/or affiliation. When seeking status, the person engages in agentic behaviour that translates into influence or control. When seeking affiliation, the individual engages in communal behaviour, trying to create bonds with the other people engaged in the interaction.

PROTOTYPICAL BEHAVIOURS

One can identify prototypical behaviours for these dimensions. For example, when behaving dominantly, a person will give information, make a suggestion, express an opinion, and set goals. Submissive behaviour is characterized by waiting for the other to act or talk first, not expressing disagreement, or letting others make plans or decisions. Sample agreeable behaviours are expressing reassurance, praising others, smiling, and laughing with others. Sample quarrelsome behaviours include not responding to another person's questions or comments, criticizing others, and withholding useful information.

FIELD STUDIES USING EVENT-CONTINGENT RECORDING

I have researched these behaviours in a series of field studies in which event-contingent recording was used. We sometimes refer to them as "diary studies." Participants are asked to record, for twenty days, information about their significant social interactions as these occur. We give participants standardized forms designed to collect information on the characteristics of the situations, the behaviours in which they and others engage, and the feelings they experience during the interactions. A significant feature of this methodology is that the data are collected in the course of individuals' daily lives, thus reflecting real interactions as they occur and minimizing retrospective biases. Our samples are comprised of working adults who are between nineteen and sixty-seven years of age and who come from a variety of occupations.

A sample form for reporting about an event would include questions concerning: (1) who was present when the interaction occurred (man, woman); (2) the role relationship with this person (supervisor, co-worker, supervisee, etc.); (3) the nature of the interpersonal relationship (acquaintance, friend, romantic partner, etc.); (4) what the person did in the interaction (listened attentively, let the other make plans, confronted the other, asked the other to do something, etc.); (5) how the person felt (on a scale from 0 to 6 – worried/anxious, happy, frustrated, etc.).

EXAMPLE OF BEHAVIOUR AND AFFECT FLUCTUATIONS

To illustrate how behaviour fluctuates, I present records of behaviour from two people we have studied. Once their data were aggregated, these people had equally high scores with regards to dominant behaviour. However, when their dominant behaviours were broken down by time of day (morning, afternoon, evening) over the twenty-day recording period, it was clear that the dominant behaviours were displayed in very different patterns. The first person (ID 18) regularly engaged in a moderate range of dominant behaviour; the second person (ID 46), in contrast, was often not dominant at all, but when this person was dominant, it was expressed in a very high range. These patterns are reproduced in Figure 2 below. Higher points indicate behaviour that was more dominant.]

The comparison of the affect data for these two people in the same twenty-day period also revealed very different patterns. In Figure 3, points greater than zero indicate positive affect; points less than zero indicate negative affect. As indicated in the figure, the first person often felt negative or neutral affect, very rarely recording positive affect. In contrast, the second person often recorded positive affect. Thus the question: how does behaviour relate to affect?

Three generalizations stem from our work (Moskowitz and Côté 1995; Côté and Moskowitz 1998; Fournier and Moskowitz 2000): (1) most people feel pleasant affect when they engage in more communal behaviour (i.e., in more frequent agreeable behaviour); people

Figure 2
Comparison between two people demonstrating equally high dominant behaviour
but in different patterns

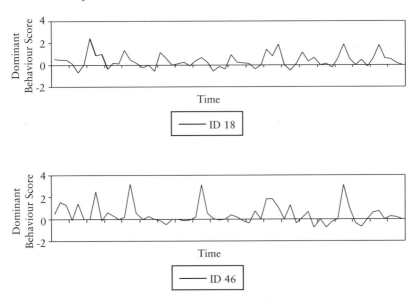

Figure 3
Comparison of affect between two people demonstrating equally high dominant
behaviour

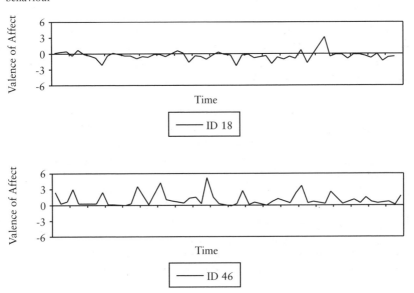

generally feel unpleasant affect when they engage in quarrelsome behaviour; (2) most people experience unpleasant affect when they engage in low agentic or submissive behaviour; (3) the highest levels of pleasant affect occur when people are highly agreeable and moderately dominant.

BEHAVIOUR AND ASSOCIATED FEELINGS DEPEND ON THE OTHER PEOPLE PRESENT

Characteristics of the role relationships between two individuals will influence the rate at which either person engages in dominant or submissive behaviour and agreeable or quarrelsome behaviour. Hierarchical roles have an influence on agentic behaviours (Moskowitz, Suh, and Desaulniers 1994b). We examined the case of people who each held three different roles; during the course of the study they had all engaged in a supervisee role, a co-worker role, and a supervisory role. Our study found that people acted differently depending upon the role played during an interaction. For example, when in the role of supervisor, they were much more agentic than when in the role of supervisee.

How people feel about their behaviour also depends on the other people present. As mentioned previously, people generally feel unpleasant affect when they are less agentic or submissive; in contrast, they feel pleasant affect when they are more agentic or moderately dominant (Fournier and Moskowitz 2000). This is true in all three of the hierarchical social relationships, but even more so when the person is in the presence of a boss. When people are with their supervisors, they enjoy being dominant, making suggestions, expressing their opinions, negotiating, and setting goals, and they feel particularly high levels of negative affect about being submissive when they are in a lower position hierarchically.

How we feel about our behaviour also depends on who we are. People who tend to be agreeable dislike engaging in quarrelsome behaviour. On the other hand, people who could be categorized as having a high level of cold-heartedness (i.e., who are thoughtless and cruel) can enjoy engaging in quarrelsome behaviour (Moskowitz and Côté 1995).

AFFECT, BEHAVIOUR, AND HEALTH CARE

Research such as the projects described in this volume has examined many examples of patient-doctor or patient-nurse relationships. But there are many other types of relationships that occur in a health care setting, such as patients' interactions with aides, occupational therapists, and rehabilitation therapists – all of whom are trying to impact on patients' behaviours and health. These people should not be forgotten in our discussions of the behaviours of health care providers. It should also be noted that no matter who the health care provider is (e.g., doctor, nurse, physical therapist) and no matter what the patient's identity is in other contexts, the patient is in a hierarchically subordinate role. Individuals in hierarchically subordinate roles tend to be more submissive and to experience negative affect in response to being submissive.

A question many health care providers ask is how to increase motivation as a means of encouraging patients to adopt the behaviours that would help them to maintain or better their health. It should be noted that adherence to medical recommendations, like adherence to other behaviours, can be presumed to fluctuate. It would be unusual for a patient to follow either all of or none of a physician's recommended procedures. Instead we can expect fluctuations in the patient's adherence to a medical or health plan; the goal of the health care profession is to reduce these fluctuations in the direction of adherence. So, ordinarily, the health care provider carefully explains what should be done, perhaps emphasizing the importance of why this should be done. But such behaviour is often perceived as dominant, further increasing the submissive role of the patient, which in turn encourages a passive response and usually engenders negative affect.

An alternative approach would be for the health care provider to support the patient's agency. For example, the health care provider can involve the patient in decision-making by helping the patient to make suggestions about how to adapt his or her lifestyle to the recommended health regime. More specifically, a health care provider might help the patient to identify when the patient will do the exercises necessary for rehabilitation, where these exercises could be done, how the patient will make adaptations in a meal schedule in order to take medications according to direction, and how these adaptations will impact on the person's routine or the routine of others in the person's household.

Some researchers have referred to this mode of involving the patient in decisions about medical care as autonomy support (Williams, Grow, Freedman, Ryan, and Deci 1996). Autonomy support is present when another individual provides a person with choices and meaningful rationales, recognizes a person's feelings and unique perspective, and refrains from pressuring a person (Reeve, Bolt, and Car 1999). The behaviours of the health care provider should increase the agentic behaviours of the patient, thereby improving the affect associated with adherence to a medical regime. Moreover, greater patient participation in decision-making and planning about the patient's situation is likely to increase the person's intrinsic motivation for adopting or maintaining behaviours that contribute to the person's health (Ryan and Deci 2000). Thus health care workers' interpersonal behaviours in dealing with the patient should serve, among other things, to increase the patient's agentic behaviour.

Zuroff, Moskowitz, and Koestner (2000) have recently proposed a model (see Figure 4) for how the interpersonal behaviours of the health care professional may contribute to more positive outcomes. Interpersonal behaviours that are agreeable and not critical and that are neither very controlling nor very submissive should contribute to the development of a helping alliance. The helping alliance should facilitate an increase in autonomous motivation, fostering the sense that the person has freely chosen the identified goals and that the choice to pursue these goals has emanated from within the person. The improved sense of autonomy should lead to cognitive changes and improved affect, thus reducing fluctuations in adherence to the medical regime.

Figure 4
Effects of interpersonal behaviour of health care professionals on care outcomes

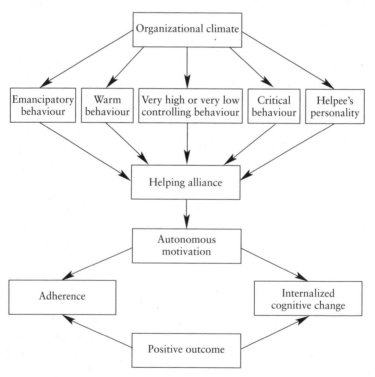

In short, health care professionals should be encouraged to engage in two kinds of behavioural strategies: (1) adopting behaviours that are relatively more communal (e.g., low on criticism, high on praise and encouragement), thereby creating an affiliative bond between the patient and the health care worker; and (2) developing a delicate balance with respect to controlling behaviours. Highly assertive behaviours on the part of health care professionals may undermine the patient's autonomy and motivation to engage in health promoting behaviours while nondirective behaviours may be perceived as unstructured and unsupportive. The health care professional should promote agentic behaviours on the part of patients by encouraging the patient to give information, make suggestions, set goals, make decisions, and otherwise determine how adherence can be maintained.

The use of these strategies should reduce the patient's sense of being in a subordinate role and contribute to the development of a collaborative alliance between patient and health care provider. This collaborative alliance may improve a patient's affect and his or her motivation to more regularly incorporate healthy behaviours for the purposes of both prevention and recovery.

I2

Methodological Challenges to Capturing Dynamical Aspects of Health Care Acquisition[1]

LAWRENCE R. LEVY, RICHARD W.J. NEUFELD, AND WEIGUANG YAO

At a psychological level, dynamics is the study of the manner in which a system, such as an individual, interacts over time with his/her environment while engaging in cognitive and emotional activity. According to physicists, dynamics examines the effects of interdependent forces on the behaviour of a system as time unfolds and the way in which the system searches for overall patterned states of stable behaviour (Barton 1994). Analogously, as individuals cognitively and emotionally transact with their surroundings on a daily basis, they quickly reach stable interpersonal, emotional, and mental states. Hence non-linear dynamical systems theory, commonly known as chaos theory, mathematically quantifies these concepts of temporality, transaction, multidimensionality and interdependence.[2] Consequently, it is a powerful tool that can greatly inform the interactive, dynamic, and temporal nature of the emotional aspects of health care.

A few decades ago, researchers from the fields of chemistry and physics demonstrated experimentally that given certain conditions, several systems

1 Sources of support for this research included a University of Western Ontario/Ontario Graduate Scholarship in Science and Technology awarded to Lawrence R. Levy and an operating grant from the Social Sciences and Humanities Research Council and an Ontario Mental Health Foundation Senior Research Fellowship awarded to Richard W.J. Neufeld.
2 Non-linear systems involve those with multiplicative terms and variables taken to higher powers, as opposed to linear systems, which have only additive terms and variables of the first power.

will exhibit highly organized behaviours that appear to be random but that are in fact strictly deterministic; they described these behaviours as being "chaotic" and "self-organized" (Prigogine and Stengers 1984). Researchers found that these complicated patterns can be predicted only in the short-term. When these systems are mathematically modelled using non-linear equations and control parameters, these coherent, complex, and novel behaviours can be simulated via computer. A control parameter is analogous to what a psychologist might refer to as an independent variable, such as an individual difference variable or an environmental constraint. In such physical and chemical systems, a control parameter refers to specific experimental manipulations that move the system through different patterned, stable states (Kelso 2000). When a continual change in a control parameter surpasses a certain threshold, the system's behaviour may change very noticeably and abruptly. For example, this process can be likened to an individual who has a very high susceptibility to the deleterious effects of psychological stress (an individual difference variable that exceeds a threshold), which can eventually result in the individual attaining an overall depressed mood (a patterned, "stable," state).

By using these mathematical models comprised of non-linear equations, it was found that as the various dimensions continuously interact with one another, the system will eventually attain a global behaviour and a specific pattern will emerge. As mentioned above, when specific thresholds in the system are surpassed, the behaviour becomes organized, and the term "self-organization" is used. In physics and chemistry, self-organization refers to a process by which a pattern emerges in an open system without specifications from the outside environment (Barton 1994). An open system is one that has dynamic interchanges with its environs. In psychology, self-organization refers to a long-term pattern (such as depressed mood state) that evolves, over time, due to the ongoing interaction of the individual with his/her environment.

Physicists stipulate that in systems that are open to interactive exchanges with their environments, unique, patterned behaviour arises due to a large number of complex interacting components (Kelso 2000). Emerging patterns are characterized by the dynamic and temporal interactions of the system's variables. Similarly, an individual who continuously interacts with his/her surroundings rapidly achieves an overall patterned mood state. Furthermore, interactions in the emotional aspects of health care are potentially so complicated that understanding may be enhanced in terms of these collective behaviours. These patterns are known as attractors and may represent static equilibria (fixed point attractors); repetitive, cyclical patterns (periodic attractors); or re-organization into complex, non-periodic patterns (chaotic attractors). It is important to note that both equilibrial and periodic patterns have long-term predictability, which aids the researcher in comprehending the future behaviours of the system. Conversely, chaotic attractors have only short-term predictability, which means that only the immediate future behaviours of the system can be predicted.

The other authors of this volume present concepts that can be aligned with non-linear dynamical systems theory: the multidimensionality of emotions, their variability over time, and their change depending upon the people involved, the situation, the type of interaction, a person's coping mechanisms, and so forth. Furthermore, these authors discuss notions of system complexity, change, predictability, interaction, and non-linearity, which are ideas espoused by this quantitative paradigm.

Non-linear dynamical systems theory is a mathematical foundation that can be utilized to better understand these complex, multifaceted, multidimensional, and interrelational aspects of emotions and health care. The richness of this approach stems from utilizing it to simulate, via computer, how various dimensions interact with one another, how these interactions unfold temporally, and how the system eventually reaches an optimal state of stability. Using high-level computational capacity, digital computers have rendered these numerical simulations possible. Moreover, these intricate and complicated health relations can harbour short-term predictability, which can aid the researcher in speculating about the future behaviour of the system.

Although these concepts are fairly novel and somewhat challenging, their use is becoming more widespread in both the natural and social sciences. In fact, although non-linear dynamical systems theory (chaos theory) has been present for several decades, its more elaborate use in science is only about a decade or so old. This is the case because the appreciable computational speed and power required to make the relevant simulations "operable" were not initially available.

TAXONOMY OF RESEARCH ARCHITECTURES

Examination of the prominent methodologies in social science research, potentially relevant to the analysis of health care acquisition, reveals a split into two major "types": the static and the dynamic (see Table 1). The static methodologies are those that are commonplace and familiar to all researchers (e.g., analysis of variance, regression analysis, and so forth). For example, when one performs an analysis of variance or inputs data into a regression equation, one is using static, linear equations to describe the relations among the variables.

Table 1
Taxonomy of relevant methodologies

	Static	*Dynamic*
Deterministic	Some decision-theory models	Non-linear dynamical systems theory (chaos theory)
Stochastic	Most univariate and multivariate statistical methods	Probabilistic process models (e.g., survival analysis)
		Stochastic non-linear dynamical systems theory

Source: Copyright 1993 American Psychological Association. Adapted, with permission of the publisher, from J.R. Busemeyer and J.T. Townsend, "Decision field theory: A dynamic-cognitive approach to decision making in an uncertain environment." *Psychological Review* 100 (1993): 433.

Since linear equations are additive, they are always easy to solve. These approaches basically take a "snapshot" of what is occurring at one specific point in time. In so doing, a researcher has in hand some statistical data and can develop some probable predictions as to what might happen if a certain variable changes. Moreover, the linear laws of cause and effect hold true, which means that small inputs into the system result in small outputs. However, the notion of time is not taken into account, and the researcher hasn't any idea of how the system temporally behaves.

In a non-linear, dynamical system, the dimensions of what one is examining (e.g., a human interaction, one's coping tendencies, one's emotions, and so forth) are entered into a simulator so that one can observe how the variables affect one another and evolve over sequential points in time. To provide an analogy, the non-linear, dynamic approach is like a movie that unfolds second by second. The researcher is the scriptwriter who can change both the outcome of the movie by varying the relations among the variables (the actors) and the relative impact that the variables (the actors) have on each other as time progresses. Such manipulations take place, of course, with an eye to titrating the system's behaviour toward maximum empirical veridicality (or, in the case of the movie, having an outcome among the actors that is as realistic as possible). In this kind of system, the linear laws of cause and effect do not hold true; small inputs to the system can result in drastically large outputs.

To examine systemic change, non-linear dynamics employs non-linear equations. However, non-linear equations are not additive and are typically difficult to solve. Moreover, the researcher can manipulate a certain parameter (individual difference variable or environmental constraint) in the system to observe how its variation affects the system at large. For example, in our laboratory, we have been investigating the non-linear dynamics of psychological stress and coping. When we manipulated, simulationally, a parameter that directly influenced the extent of one's cognitive appraisal of the level of stress in the environment, the stability of the system drastically changed and reconstituted itself into a new organization. The quantitative change in just one parameter (individual difference variable) caused the entire system to exhibit a totally novel form of behaviour that could not have been discovered or predicted otherwise. Hence a chaotic attractor (a complex, non-periodic pattern) emerged, which may have important implications for researchers' and clinicians' understanding of psychological stress and coping processes.

THE PREVENTION AND EARLY INTERVENTION PROGRAM FOR PSYCHOSES (PEPP)

The following example illustrates a dynamical model of care. In Ontario, Canada, the PEPP program is attempting to reach people who are prone to schizophrenia in order to encourage them to seek treatment before the onset of the disorder. Drs Ashok Malla and Ross Norman and their collaborators at the London Health Sciences Centre have launched an advertising campaign in schools that presents some of the main symptoms of the disease – such as having delusions, hallucinations, and disorganized speech and choosing to be extremely socially isolated. With this "ad campaign," the researchers are hoping that friends will encourage individuals who manifest these behaviours and symptoms to seek immediate treatment.

The challenge is to reach genuinely vulnerable individuals and to have them treated as soon as possible. To do that, it is necessary to maximize the number of individuals correctly identified as needing intervention. The question arises as to how to refine the criteria so that the number of "hits" is maximized. Moreover, it would be beneficial to be aware of the time frame within which to enlist ill individuals into the program. One can be aided in refining criteria and time frames by capitalizing on what one knows about the dynamics involved in this process-oriented system and about the variables pertaining to this disorder that interact over time.

Based upon the qualitative and quantitative data at hand, the main dimensions of the system are defined. In this case, six dimensions were chosen, as presented in Table 2. These are the components that are temporally and dynamically interacting with one another. For purposes

Table 2
Prototypical variables for a dynamical model of care acquisition

$Y_1(t)$	Level of health-threatening signals (exogenous and endogenous)
$Y_2(t)$	Level of factors adversely affecting efficiency of health-promoting/care-acquiring behaviours
$Y_3(t)$	Efficiency of health-promoting/care-acquiring behaviours
$Y_4(t)$	Actual level of health-promoting activity
$Y_5(t)$	Sensitivity of factors adversely affecting efficiency of health-promoting behaviours ($Y_2(t)$) to sources of adverse effects (disrupting properties of $Y_1(t)$; negative experiences surrounding $Y_4(t)$)
$Y_6(t)$	Responsivity of health-promoting activity ($Y_4(t)$) to health-threatening signals ($Y_1(t)$)

Note: All dimensions include a *t* (time) because once the system is put in motion, the results vary along a time span.

of a simplified example, the control parameters (individual difference variables and/or environmental constraints) involved in such a system will not be considered.

$Y_1(t)$, the level of health-threatening signals, relates both to the symptomatology of the disease (endogenous factors) and to environmental (exogenous) factors that can come into play (e.g., health-adverse economic, climactic, or even political disruptions). It is in $Y_2(t)$, levels of factors countering health-promoting/care-acquiring behaviours, that emotions tentatively come into play. These are the factors that may perturb individuals' compliance with a physician's advice or interfere with their seeking treatment. They are emotions that might block cognitive efficiency concerning what one knows one should be doing versus what one chooses to do. An example would be the social smoker who knows that smoking is bad for his/her health but chooses to continue smoking.

$Y_3(t)$ relates to the efficiency of health-maintaining/promoting activities (e.g., the extent to which the therapeutic compliance actually pays off in terms of better health). $Y_4(t)$ is the actual level of health-promoting activity. $Y_5(t)$ is the sensitivity of factors adversely affecting the efficiency of health-promoting behaviours [$Y_2(t)$] to sources of adverse effects [$Y_1(t)$] and to certain aspects of $Y_4(t)$ (e.g., frustrating consequences of health-promoting efforts). $Y_6(t)$ is the responsivity of health-promoting activity [$Y_4(t)$] to health-threatening signals [$Y_1(t)$].

Once these dimensions have been chosen, each is defined by a non-linear equation expressing the direction and speed of its change at any point in time with reference to the other dimensions of the system. The construction of each equation is guided as much as possible by

observational and empirical data. The parameters (individual difference variables and/or environmental constraints) and constants of the
equational system are then selected. The resulting non-linear equations
are subsequently used to set the dynamics in motion. These equations
are based on the theoretical principles of non-linear dynamical systems
theory (chaos theory).

Once the system is set up, one can start examining how the system
unfolds as time evolves. One can observe how all of these variables
constantly interact with each other and how their effects on each other
impact on their numerical values in the non-linear, dynamical system.
These values constantly fluctuate between being high and low; thus
these different levels operate in tandem. This is why such a set-up is
called a highly coupled, interactive, dynamical system.

As the dynamics of the system unfold, one notices changes over time
in each of the variables. This feature of non-linear dynamical modelling
makes it an invaluable and informative tool. One can observe how the
value of one variable changes in relation to the values of the other
variables. Moreover, one can glimpse the reasons for these interactions
by referring back to the original equations. From these observations,
interesting, new avenues of research on our specific topic are unveiled,
as are new ways of thinking about it. Further, one can be alerted to
the strategic times for potential intervention and remedial responses.
For example, in the PEPP program, these times could indicate when to
effectively recruit ill individuals for the program. Once the research
has been done, we can reintegrate our findings into the system and
again look at how it unfolds as time evolves. Most importantly, the
variables that change discontinuously are often the most information-
ally meaningful for the research domain of interest. As well, a bifurcation in the system could occur, in which there is an abrupt change
in a system's long-term pattern (attractor) at a critical value of a
control parameter (individual difference variable and/or environmental
constraint). As alluded to earlier, a control parameter is any systemic
component that operates as a primary agent of change. At the point
of bifurcation, the elements of the system's old pattern come into
contact with one another in novel ways and make new connections,
resulting in a new overall behaviour or state. A small change in a
particular control parameter can initiate this major phase shift, with
remarkable repercussions for the entire system. Stated simply, due to
the high level of an individual difference variable (for example, an
individual's very high degree of reactivity to psychological stressors)
and its interaction with other factors (such as the individual's low
coping activity, low cognitive efficiency, and very high emotional

arousal), the individual may find him/herself "locked" in an attractor state (such as depressed mood).

A question arises as to why all of these variables are interacting and affecting one another. The answer lies in non-linear dynamical systems theory, by which any system that is being "disturbed" will seek to come back to an "attractor" – i.e., to an equilibrium point (fixed point), periodic behaviour, or quasi-periodic behaviour (perturbed cyclic behaviour). However, the system may reconstitute itself into a new organization, termed "self-organization," such as a chaotic attractor (an apparently random configuration that, in actuality, has no random components). Hence non-linear systems tend to converge to stable behaviour over time. What is interesting for us as health care researchers is the opportunity to see just how the system will unfold over time to reach that point of stability. In addition, as mentioned above, in some cases the system will evolve into a totally novel mode of stability, such as a chaotic attractor, that may give the researcher some new insight into the system.

We can also see how two or three variables are linked to one another. In principle, with this knowledge we can estimate the relative presence of health-promoting behaviour. If this behaviour is deemed deficient, the analysis potentially discloses avenues of intervention. A variable comprising a nexus for pervasive influence of other variables in the system may be indicated. Such a variable, for example, would be one pertaining to cognitive efficiency. In other words, with a non-linear, dynamical system, one can evaluate how one variable is affecting a multiplicity of other variables. Throughout, one can observe how the altered system stabilizes, and this new stability can greatly inform the researcher as to the new behaviour being evinced, including its health-promoting properties. In this way, the formal-systems perspective could ideally inform intervention in a unique way, ensuring maximum impact.

It is important to note that even complicated, potentially chaotic systems, such as the one delineated above, have short-term predictability. Although the complexity of the system is determined by the evolution of the non-linear equations, it can be quantified via several numerical indices (Neufeld 1999). Unfortunately, these diagnostic markers are beyond the scope of this chapter. As mentioned above, one is able to predict how the aforementioned system will behave in both the short- and long-term, depending upon the values of the control parameters (individual difference variables and/or environmental constraints). This forecast, in turn, can also inform the researcher involved in programs such as PEPP of the best windows of opportunity for remedial intervention in an individual's care.

PSYCHOLOGICAL STRESS AND COPING

The above illustration is but one example of a system and the variables that compose it. Another system that has been developed pertains to psychological stress and coping (Neufeld 1999). Table 3 lists the six dimensions that were employed. This model is presented merely to offer insight into the flexibility and versatility of non-linear dynamical systems theory.

It is important to acknowledge that stress researchers have long beckoned for what is offered by a non-linear, dynamical systems approach to stress and coping. As early as 1952, Lazarus, Deese, and Osler noted that an integrated, theoretical framework of the effects of psychological stress upon cognitive and behavioural performance was necessary and that such a framework must consider individual differences, impairment and improvement of performance, and the influence of different environmental situations.

Folkman and Lazarus (1985) have stated that "the essence of stress, coping, and adaptation is change ... Therefore, unless we focus on change, we cannot learn how people come to manage stressful events and conditions" (150). Lazarus (2001) reiterates the same notion, emphasizing that psychological stress is "change in time" and "flux." Moreover, a person is a complex, integrated system that manages stressful transactions with the environment and that is being shaped and changed by these transactions on an ongoing basis (Lazarus 1990). The use of non-linear dynamical systems theory is thus an attempt to develop a theoretical modus operandi for predicting change.

This prototype seeks to present the reciprocal influences, multicomponentiality, and interdependencies among stress, coping, and other variables, such as cognitive appraisal (see Table 3). The theoretical framework is partly an outgrowth of a prior mathematical model of psychological stress and schizophrenia (Neufeld and Nicholson 1991; Nicholson and Neufeld 1992). The layout of variables applies to a "decisional control" form of coping in a stressful situation (Lees and Neufeld 1999; Morrison, Neufeld, and Lefebvre 1988). Employing that kind of coping mechanism involves cognitive activity since a person will try to predict (using "predictive judgments") the level of threat entailed by various choice responses. He/she will tend to use the least threatening and most efficient option, according to his/her judgment. Thus cognitive activity plays a central role in navigating through a stressful situation in order to reach the most advantageous resolution. As mentioned earlier, in our laboratory, it has been demonstrated that as the perceived efficacy of this effortful cognitive activity

Table 3
Stress and coping: Six dimensions of a prototypical, interactive, dynamical system

$Y_1(t)$	Level of collective external stressor properties, accessible to decisional control
$Y_2(t)$	Level of stress arousal – should increase in response to certain external stressor properties
$Y_3(t)$	Level of cognitive efficiency – as stress arousal increases, cognitive efficiency potentially decreases
$Y_4(t)$	Level of coping activity in the form of decisional control (e.g., formulating and implementing threat-minimizing predictive judgments bearing on options for negotiating a multifaceted stressing situation)
$Y_5(t)$	Degree to which the level of stress arousal ($Y_2(t)$) is sensitive to disruption associated with $Y_1(t)$ and mentally taxing properties of $Y_4(t)$
$Y_6(t)$	Responsivity of the coping activity level ($Y_4(t)$) to the level of external stressor properties ($Y_1(t)$)

Note: All dimensions include a *t* (time) because once the system is put in motion, the results vary along a time span.

increases, the entire system is propelled into a completely new organization of behaviour, termed "self-organization," and a chaotic attractor emerges.

The prototype puts into play six dimensions that interact with one another in time, making it a dynamic, time-dependent model. The dimensions are the levels of external stressors, stress arousal, cognitive efficiency, coping activity, and dynamic stress and coping resiliences. It should be noted that each level is an aggregate or summary index of the respective dimension. Moreover, the six dimensions are quantified by the implementation of non-linear differential equations. A differential equation is a proposed mathematical law that involves the rates of change of various dependent variables with respect to one independent variable: time (Spiegel 1967).

Once the dimensions have been chosen, the next step is to define certain parameters (individual difference variables and/or environmental constraints) that are relevant to each dimension and that should be included in the numerical equations. For example, when looking at the level of the external stressor properties ($Y_1(t)$), the equation appropriates three parameters: (1) the degree to which the environment tends to propagate the stressor properties in the absence of countering influences, (2) the extent to which coping activities and cognitive efficiency can diminish such properties, and (3) the extent to which the level of stressor properties tends to increase more when it is relatively low and less when it is already relatively high.

Applying the Model

Applying such a model to human behaviour is surely more complex than applying it in fields such as chemistry and physics, where, for instance, self-organization has been empirically observed. For example, if one were to apply the model to fluid dynamics, one would base the parameters and constants on direct and precise measurements. By measuring these naturally occurring environmental variations, values would be obtained that could be substituted into the equations. In the field of behavioural sciences, the numerically computed paths would be based on reasonable values one would have ascertained through observations, be they quantitative or qualitative. Thus one would put the system through a test run with what could be termed "guesstimates." Examining how the system path unfolds, one would refine the guesstimates to reach optimal correspondence between model-predicted and observed dimension trajectories. Once that had been done, one could set the system in motion and learn from it how all the dimensions vary over time and impact one another. Moreover, using computational manipulation of the system's parameters (individual difference variables and/or environmental constraints), one could observe the system's changes in patterned, stable states.

Again, we refer to the work done in our laboratory. We have found that, simulationally, cognitive efficiency $(Y_3(t))$ can modify both the level of stressor properties $(Y_1(t))$ and the coping activity $(Y_4(t))$. On the other hand, cognitive efficiency $(Y_3(t))$ increases with a reduction in stress arousal $(Y_2(t))$. Additionally, the degree to which one activates cognitive appraisal of coping efficacy has emerged as the most change-facilitating construct in the model. The accentuation of this psychological construct causes the entire system to restabilize itself, and the system emerges as more highly and intricately ordered.

Researchers in our laboratory continue to fine-tune and empirically validate this system, which is behaviourally principled with respect to psychological stress and coping. For example, we have embarked on the process of coupling some of the variables and have found that the process leads to a more robust system. With coupling, we have discovered that the responsivity of coping activity to changes in stressor levels $(Y_6(t))$ can be influenced by the appraised coping efficacy. When coping responsiveness is directly informed by assessed "returns on coping" (as operationalized mathematically), adaptability of the system at large evidently increases. For example, greater elevations in cumulative stressor levels $(Y_1(t))$ can be absorbed without disruption of the eventual system-wide return to an equilibrium-attractor state (fixed point attractor).

CONCLUSION

Non-linear, dynamical systems such as the ones presented above in general rather than mathematical terms can serve researchers who want to test some hypotheses relating to emotions, interpersonal behaviours, and health. The simulations that can be set in motion are launched from the domain of empirical observation and can be used to form predictions concerning what data should be collected next and what collective patterns (overall behaviours or mood states) ought to form.

Many of this book's authors could apply non-linear dynamical systems modelling to their research endeavours in order to address issues in emotional health such as multidimensionality, interdependence, transaction, and temporality.

Many computer simulation programs are available for those who would like to use them to advance their research and to refine a research agenda pertaining to emotions and health. There are a multitude of specialists in the field who can support endeavours such as translating verbal arguments into quantitative dynamics. Researchers should seize the opportunities made available to them to use these tools to serve their research projects. To our knowledge, they remain the only route to gaining a rigorous theoretical foothold on the complexities of reciprocal influences among variables across time (Staddon 1984).

In order to use non-linear dynamical modelling, it is strongly suggested that assistance be sought from a person who is familiar with the software available – e.g., programs such as Phaser (Kocak 1989) and Chaos Data Analyzer: Professional Version (Sprott and Rowlands 1995) – and who is knowledgeable about this quantitative theory, including assumptions concerning the data at hand, necessary for valid inferences. Once variables have been chosen, they can be entered into a computer program, such as Chaos Data Analyzer: Professional Version, that can help characterize the nature of the system involved and possibly aid in setting up prediction equations pertaining to future values of the system dimensions.

It is recommended that the following three steps be taken: (1) set up the system with the qualitative and quantitative data available, which includes devising a set of non-linear equations with appropriate control parameters; (2) determine how the system operates as time unfolds (using available software such as Matlab, Waterloo Maple, or Phaser) and fine-tune as necessary; (3) monitor how the software simulations express themselves when applied to actual data, using numerical diagnostic software such as Chaos Data Analyzer: Professional Version.

Overall, the utility of a non-linear, dynamical systems approach for health care researchers appears indispensable. Through the use of computer simulations, the ability to model the temporal dynamics of specific emotional disorders enables, potentially, the effective and timely targeting of remedial interventions. Moreover, researchers' understanding of the interactive, multidimensional, and dynamic nature of acquiring health care can only be enhanced by incorporating such a novel paradigm. By paying attention to the multiple factors involved in health care acquisition, how they change over time, and what functional or dysfunctional outcome the system (individual who interacts with his/her environment) eventually reaches, researchers and clinicians in health care will be better informed about their patients' decisions regarding the treatment of their emotional disorders.

13

Outcomes in Health Care: Motivation, Measures, and Drivers at the Population Level

TERRENCE MONTAGUE

In the biomedical and pharmaceutical domains, breakthroughs have been made possible by the development of a solid theoretical understanding not only of health and diseases, but also of medical and pharmaceutical interventions. Breakthroughs have also been supported by a relentless quest for innovation and by extensive empirical testing of the efficacy of any new diagnostic or therapeutic intervention. I contend that a similar approach will have to be developed in the more human aspects of care like emotion and interpersonal processes if these are to become integral parts of health service research and practice. In this chapter, I first review some recent Canadian experiences with population-level measurements of the effectiveness of medical and pharmaceutical interventions. Measurement is an important and integral part of the agenda since measures at the population level can be useful in determining the "what" and the "how" in order to eventually resolve the "why" of our current practices, all of which may allow for improvements in practices and outcomes. I then introduce a model to assess and reduce the gap that may exist between current practices and evidence-based, efficacious treatments.

MEASUREMENT AS A VALUE SYSTEM

In looking at the objective of developing a research agenda in the health domain, one must consider the professional diversity of the people involved – some have graduated from schools of management; others are physicians, nurses, or health care researchers; some have backgrounds in psychology and others in marketing. All have an interest in, and contributions to make to, the health agendas.

Looking at my own path through medical school, I must say that its teachings did not include anything about institutional ethics, institutional theory, or organizational behaviour. I still don't know very much about these domains, although I do know that they are all relevant to measuring and explaining some of the gaps and challenges in our current health system.

Seeking to know more, I spoke to an expert on ethics in the health management field. Her name is Sister Nuala Kenny. She is a nun and a physician. Presently, she is a professor of paediatrics and the founding director of the Centre of Bioethics Education and Research at Dalhousie University. In Sister Kenny's template of ethical institutional behaviour, measurement represents an important value system founded on criteria that are durable and transparent, and upon which we are prepared to act. And, when actions are taken, it is with "all cards on the table" and in response to evidence of sufficiently high quality to be likely feasible, and representative, in real-world settings.

There are many means of measurement in the health sciences. Figure 1 below illustrates several commonly used measurement designs presented along an inference continuum, where the degree of certainty that can be safely assumed about the cause of the results ranges from speculative (on the left) to firm (on the right). When measuring, we are well served to keep in mind these different levels of evidence, or quantitative degrees of certainty, based on how much causal inference can be assumed from any study's methodology.

As indicated in Figure 1, large randomized controlled trials provide a very high degree of certainty of result. This doesn't mean, however, that truth can't be discovered from anecdotal observations, but rather that there is a high risk of bias in assigning cause based on a single observation. For example, if a practitioner in the coronary care unit of a hospital who is treating a patient suffering from potentially fatal ventricular dysrhythmia successfully administers a drug associated with the return of normal rhythm and the preservation of life, a natural inference is: The drug saved the patient's life. However, if the practitioner then decides to administer the same drug to a hundred consecutive patients with the same cardiac complication, and more patients die than live, what is the correct conclusion? Does the drug cause more harm than good?

The above example serves to show the need for robust, carefully designed, large, randomized, controlled trials, as these reduce the risk of systematic and play-of-chance errors in process and interpretation. The happy reality is that the widespread adoption of large, simple, clinical trials has resulted in a situation in which, for many disease

Figure 1
Measurement as a value system: A motivating ethic

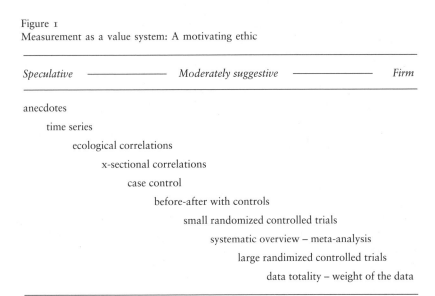

| *Speculative* | ———————— | *Moderately suggestive* | ———————— | *Firm* |

anecdotes

    time series

        ecological correlations

           x-sectional correlations

             case control

                before-after with controls

                    small randomized controlled trials

                        systematic overview – meta-analysis

                          large randimized controlled trials

                              data totality – weight of the data

states, clinicians and researchers know what works and what doesn't. The concomitant reality that we are still struggling with is: Can we make efficacious therapies work for more people? This question underscores the very real imperative to know the institutional ethical framework on which decisions are based. Challenges arise because many stakeholders are involved, and each uses its own frame of reference. The approach that I have increasingly used in my practice is to apply the Kenny formula: Is there an evidence base for the decision? What is the level of causal inference? Are all the decision proponents also operational within another value system that is durable and believed in enough to be acted upon? And are actions transparent, with all the cards on the table? This approach has been useful in developing the care gap model presented next.

BEST CARE VERSUS USUAL CARE: THE CARE GAP

My colleagues and I, over the past ten years, have been working on outcomes research along a continuum of care. What we have repeatedly encountered is what we have come to call the care gap (Montague 1999). By this term we mean: If best care is defined as proven, efficacious therapy, and if usual care is defined as what audit and survey data show is the level of efficacious care actually being provided to the whole population at risk, the care gap is any deficit between the two.

In other words, robust research has defined what best care is for many disease states by identifying tests with acceptable predictive value and therapies that are producing more good than harm. But, at the societal level, there is a discrepancy between the concept of best care and what is actually being delivered on a daily basis. Many people at risk – those who could benefit from proven therapies – are not bene-fiting from them. This is the care gap: Best care does not equal usual care for the whole population at risk.

In fact, about fifteen years ago, Peter Tugwell, then at McMaster University, theorized much of what subsequently has been confirmed by practice and outcomes audits (Tugwell, Bennett, Sackett, and Haynes 1985). He and a group of his colleagues observed that clinical trials were rapidly becoming able to recognize whether care was more beneficial than harmful or the converse. This was particularly salient for the cardiovascular diseases, which were, and remain, the number one killers in our society. Tugwell et al. wondered: What is preventing population health outcomes from looking like the results promised from the clinical trials? They predicted that the principal causes of care gaps in population health were likely to be poor diagnosis of treatable disease, poor prescription of proven therapies for the target diseases, poor concordance with prescribed therapy, and poor access to that therapy. Any one, or combination, of these factors could contribute to suboptimal outcomes in the whole population at risk. They were right.

From the viewpoint of patients, it is immaterial which single cause, or combination of causes, is operative in creating the care gap; the end result is the same. There is no chance of achieving the improved out-come promised by the efficacious therapy in the absence of the therapy. From the perspective of professionals, however, it is important to mea-sure care gaps, to point to their causes and consequences, and most importantly to reduce them.

Measuring the Care Gap

The Clinical Quality Improvement Network (cqin), based at the Uni-versity of Alberta, was formed about ten years ago. It is a group of physicians, pharmacists, nurses, and other health care workers and researchers who, motivated by the widespread existence of the care gap across many diseases, decided to work toward closing it (Tsuyuki, Teo, Ikuta, Bay, Greenwood, and Montague 1994; cqin investigators 1995, 1996). Next, I present a few research programs designed to achieve this objective.

Care Gap: Prescription

The CQIN's research has repeatedly shown that large proportions of at-risk populations do not receive proven therapy, even in tertiary care centres. Table 1 below displays representative patterns of practice data for the treatment of, and the hospital mortality resulting from, heart attacks, a disease for which there are numerous proven therapies. Note that within the care gap for each drug therapy, there is a consistently greater gap for older patients – a biologically counterintuitive observation that has been measured in almost all similar practice pattern audits, irrespective of disease or geography (Tsuyuki et al. 1994; CQIN investigators 1995, 1996).

Aspirin, beta blockers, and thrombolysis are all proven therapies that save lives. Why, then, does this prescription gap persist? And why is it that the results presented in Table 1 reveal such a greater gap for older patients? These are questions with no simple or singular causal attribution.

One might hope that practices have changed since the above data were collected. Indeed, there have been some closures of gaps. However, the most recent data from the Improving Cardiac Outcomes in Nova Scotians (ICONS) study confirm persisting gaps in many proven heart attack therapies (Cox 1999; Sidel, Ryan, and Nemis-White 1998). And a large recent survey of general practitioners, internists, and cardiologists revealed qualitatively similar, although quantitatively smaller, gaps for all of the therapies studied in the earlier CQIN analyses (Taylor, Teo, Cox, Alter, Ashton, Tremblay, and Montague 2000a; Taylor, Teo, Tymchak, Cox, Alter, Ashton, Tremblay, and Montague 2000b). Moreover, the survey results revealed persistent underprescription of the proven therapies for older patients (Taylor et al. 2000b).

Table 1
Care gap: Prescription (heart attack treatment)

Drug therapy (*p < 0.0001) (n = 2,070)	Of patients < 70, % receiving the therapy	Of patients > 70, % receiving the therapy
Aspirin*	83	65
Beta blockers*	52	33
Thrombolysis*	34	16
Hospital mortality*	7	25

Source: Copyright 1994 Chest. Adapted, with permission of the publisher, from R.T. Tsuyuki et al., "Mortality risk and patterns of practice in 2070 patients with acute myocardial infarction 1987–92: The relative importance of age, sex and medical therapy," Chest 105 (1994): 1,688, 1,699.

Care Gap: Compliance

A second major contributor to the care gap is less than optimal compliance with proven therapies, even when they are prescribed. My colleagues and I have come to view this problem as a lack of concordance between caregivers (doctors/nurses/pharmacists) and care receivers (patients/families) in how they balance the seesaw of risk and benefit analysis for a given disease and its treatment (Sidel et al. 1998). The parties are not in concordance in their thinking and in their interpretations of the evidence, and this results in a lack of conviction concerning the need for persistence in adopting, and thus poor compliance with, prescribed therapies.

Compliance is a problem in many diseases and with many therapies. On average, the highest rates of compliance are with immunosuppressant drugs, which are essential to controlling the threat of rejection of transplanted organs. Nonetheless, in my experience, compliance even with this life-saving therapy is less than 100 per cent! In clinical medicine, on a day-to-day basis, the matter of compliance is becoming more and more of a concern because of the aging population and the consequent age-related increase in chronic diseases such as arthritis, osteoporosis, atherosclerosis, and dementia. Our repeated internal analyses (Sidel et al. 1998) have confirmed averages of about 50 per cent for patient compliance, or persistence, with proven therapies – such as hypertension and cardiovascular risk reduction – one year after the inception of therapy.

The causes of non-compliance appear to be multiple and complex, suggesting their improvement will be difficult. However, improvement is not impossible if some of the processes that are used in clinical trials can be effectively transferred to entire populations at risk. In the recently published results from one trial, the Simvastatin/Enalapril Coronary Atherosclerosis Trial (SCAT), compliance with a primary lipid lowering therapy was more than 95 per cent over the trial's five-year duration (Teo, Burton, Buller, Plante, Catellier, Tymchak, Dzavik, Taylor, Yokoyama, and Montague 2000). In contrast, as indicated above and based on our experience, the expected real-world population compliance would be only 50 to 60 per cent at six months (Sidel et al. 1998). The SCAT measurements empirically demonstrate that it is possible to reach much higher compliance rates.

Care Gap: Diagnosis

Of the four components of the care gap, the least defined by robust measurement is suboptimal diagnosis, in part because it is so difficult to reliably measure in many disease states. For example, the real prevalence or total population of people with asymptomatic diseases is uncertain. Present estimates suggest that the diagnostic rate for people suffering from such disease processes is about 35 per cent. This means that two people out of three who have an asymptomatic disease don't even know they do. It is not probable that these people will seek medical care when they don't even know they have a disease. And, if they do know, another impediment may be the presence of various definitions of what constitutes a diagnostic threshold for a given disease.

If osteoporosis is considered representative of a chronic disease, our recent estimates of the burden of illness and diagnostic rates around osteoporosis suggest that there is a large window of opportunity to close the care gap. Of a total population of 1.4 million people in Canada with osteoporosis, we have estimated that approximately 1.1 million are seen by an MD for some reason but that only 480,000 are diagnosed with this often asymptomatic, but ultimately risky, disease of the elderly. In comparison, the diagnostic rates for patients with symptomatic heart disease – for example, for patients with angina or heart attacks – likely approach 100 per cent.

Care Gap: Access

Restricted access to health care is a reality in Canada even though we speak of universality, or unrestricted access, as being a dominant principle and watchword of our current care paradigm. The access component of the care gap is illustrated to some degree by reviewing the provincial formulary listing decisions for innovative new drugs that recently received a "notice of compliance" for sale in Canada from the federal minister of health. No province is providing rapid, universal, unrestricted access to, and remuneration for, all new medications. The province giving the highest rate of recent access to the new drugs studied was Quebec. Ontario is the province in which the time between the submission of a new drug for listing and its granting is the longest, almost 50 percent greater than the national average of 361 days.

A second level of impaired access, at least for the elderly, is the increasing adoption of province/patient co-payments for formulary-listed medications. Not unlike the variation in listing status itself, there is great variability among the provinces in the absolute amounts of patient co-payments required for similar medications. As evidenced recently by the increased co-payment requirement in Quebec, there is no doubt that for patients on fixed, or limited, incomes having to pay out of their own pockets is another impediment to receiving potentially beneficial medications.

The primary driver for restricting formulary access is, presumably, the desire to reduce drug costs in provincial budgets. The Achilles heel of this restrictive policy, however, is that although the cost-saving goals of restricting formulary access may be realized for the drug budget, they are often offset by increased health system costs incurred in other budgets when adverse clinical events are not prevented because proven therapy is not used.

This has been repeatedly shown by numerous studies conducted in the US (Montague, Sidel, Erhardt, Nakhlé, Caron, Croteau, Kader, Haket, Skilton, and McLeod 1997). In fact, the weight of evidence from these published studies is overwhelmingly consistent on three points: (1) the elderly are disproportionately targeted in restrictive formulary policies; (2) the intended goal is often achieved – targeted drug component costs go down; and (3) the intended cost savings are frequently offset when the whole health system is considered, both in clinical and costs terms – that is, the net systems costs are greater.

It would appear that unless a health policy restricts something that, on average, produces more harm than good, the policy will produce unintended adverse outcomes (Montague et al. 1997). The reasons for this phenomenon are still not completely certain. One obvious interpretation is that individual doctors and patients make, on average, better use of all available evidence and value systems in deciding what is likely to produce therapeutic benefit than do formulary policy committees.

In summary, the challenge in correcting restricted access's contribution to the care gap seems to be to alter the current climate, in which payers focus on minimizing overuse of medications in order to ensure appropriate use for everybody at risk who could benefit.

Care Gap: Overall

Speaking of care gaps to an audience of 135 physicians and nurses in Atlantic Canada, I asked them if they felt care gaps were real. Ninety-three per cent felt they were. Then I asked their opinion of what weight they would give to the various contributing causes of the care gap. For them suboptimal prescription and compliance were dominant factors. Interestingly, when I posed the same question to a lay audience of Kiwanis Club members, they were unanimous in picking restricted access as the most important contributing cause. Obviously, how one views the care gap is determined by one's role in the provision and reception of health care. For example, the feeling that restricted access is a large problem for people, if widespread in the lay public's mind, may underlie the consistent perceptions of declining quality of health care reported by successive samplings of public opinion. Our understanding of this possible relationship may benefit from further research.

CLOSING THE CARE GAP WITH PARTNERSHIP AND MEASUREMENT

To paraphrase the German writer Goethe, "It's no longer enough to just know, we must do." The CQIN group adopted this philosophy. Its aim was to close the care gap, not just to measure it. The CQIN recipe was to create a broad-based, grass roots partnership whose members would measure and analyse practices and outcomes. These outcomes were circulated among the members, and, based on this feedback, new interventions were proposed and implemented. In turn, new baseline measurements were conducted, resulting in the circulation of additional, revised data. The process thus became a continuous quality improvement loop.

The magic in the recipe is the continuous improvement in practices and outcomes based on repeated measurement and data feedback. This has been ascribed to the Hawthorne, or trial, effect – the underlying cause of which remains obscure seventy years after its discovery. It appears, however, ubiquitous in medicine. And perhaps this is not surprising if one considers that some type of altruism is probably one cause of the Hawthorne effect. Even overworked and burnt-out physicians and nurses still want to do a good job. And, if they can be consistently provided with measures of gaps in diagnosis, prescription, and compliance, they will act upon them to improve the situation. The care gaps measurements thus become a motivator, a stimulus to do better.

Does the recipe work? The answer is yes! For example, a study conducted at the University of Alberta hospitals over many years showed that using the model of repeated measurement and feedback with the aim of increasing the utilization of proven drugs and decreasing the use of non-proven drugs in heart attack management was very, and continuously, successful (Sidel et al. 1998). One of the major outcomes of the project was a significant decrease in in-hospital patient mortality. In 1987, the year the study began, the in-hospital mortality rate for patients over seventy-eight years of age was 35 per cent; it had declined to 17 per cent by 1992. For younger patients, the rate remained approximately the same (7 per cent in 1987; 6 per cent in 1992) (Sidel et al. 1998).

THE IMPROVING CARDIAC OUTCOMES IN NOVA SCOTIANS (ICONS) PROJECT

The most mature disease management project in which Merck Frosst is currently conducting measurements is the ICONS study (Cox 1999; Sidel et al. 1998). In our concept, disease or health management is defined as: a focused application of health resources to achieve a desired outcome. More specifically, our Patient Health Management (PHM) projects measure some or all of the major contributors to the care gap – that is, poor diagnosis, poor prescription, poor compliance, and poor access – and utilize repeated feedback of these measurements to continuously drive the Hawthorne effect.

At Merck Frosst, particularly in PHM, the accent is on patients in the dynamic continuum from health to disease and back to health. PHM is considered optimal management because it fosters not only trial-proven treatment, but treatment that is comprehensive, seamless from institutions to the community, and respectful of retaining the power deriving from the individual decision-making covenant between caregiver and care receiver. As with the CQIN projects, the most important facets of the PHM programs' success are the broad partnerships that develop around the common goals of best care for the most people at the best cost and the commitment to continuous measurement and feedback of all outcomes and processes. In the ICONS study, the focus is on cardiovascular diseases, still the most clinically and fiscally burdensome diseases in our modern society. The target population is all patients with cardiovascular diseases in Nova Scotia.

Ensuring meaningful changes for the whole target population requires that the steering committee be very broad based and truly representative of the community. Thus the ICONS steering committee has a large membership, including: (1) patients and patient advocates (Heart and Stroke Foundation of Nova Scotia); (2) community providers (physicians, nurses, pharmacists); (3) government officials (Nova Scotia Department of Health); (4) health care industry officials (Merck Frosst Canada Ltd); (5) service providers (information technicians); and (6) academics (medicine, pharmacy, nursing, continuing health education).

As predicted from earlier studies, the emerging ICONS data for all hospitals and communities in Nova Scotia suggest that the processes of measurement and feedback are working. For example, when community and in-hospital prescription patterns for lipid lowering drug use among acute ischemic syndrome patients were compared over the first two years of the project, it was revealed that evidence-based, appropriate use had increased more than 50 per cent in both settings.

OTHER PHM PROJECTS

Presently, we are involved in several other major disease management projects across Canada, and there are plans for others. In all the projects, the vision is the same: the best health for the most people at the best cost. Many questions, however, remain to be answered: (1) Are care gaps inevitable? (2) Is PHM the best model for improving care/outcomes? (3) Will health stakeholders and governments buy in? (4) Will the model guide policy decisions and reduce restrictive component management? (5) Will the research and development community buy in? Time, a lot of dedicated effort, and a lot of robust measurements will provide the answers. As mentioned at the outset of this paper, these are likely prerequisites as well for innovative research and practice developments in the more human aspects of care.

References

ACSI webpage: http://www.bus.umich.edu/research/nqrc/acsi.htm. Accessed May 2000.

Aday, L.A., and R. Andersen. 1975. *Access to medical care.* Ann Arbor, MI: Health Administration Press.

– R. Andersen, and G.V. Fleming. 1980. *Health care in the U.S.: Equitable for whom?* Beverly Hills, CA: Sage Publications.

Aiken, L.H., C.E. Lewis, J. Craig, R.C. Mendenhall, R.J. Blendon, and D.E. Rogers. 1979. "The contribution of specialists to the delivery of primary care." *New England Journal of Medicine* 300: 1,363–70.

– and D.M. Sloane. 1997. "Effects of organizational innovation in AIDS care on burnout among hospital nurses." *Work & Occupation* 24: 453–77.

– D.M. Sloane, and J. Sochalski. 1998. "Hospital organization and outcomes." *Quality in Health Care* 7: 222–6.

– S.P. Clarke, D.M. Sloane, J. Sochalski, and J. Silber. 2002. "Hospital nurse staffing and patient mortality, nurse burnout and job dissatisfaction." *Journal of the American Medical Association* 288: 1,987–93.

Alberta Association of Registered Nurses. 2001. "Nursing shortage." Available at http://www.nurses.ab.ca/issues/shortage.html. Accessed 25 May 2001.

Alberta Health. 1994. "Healthy Albertans living in a healthy Alberta: A three-year business plan." Edmonton: Alberta Health.

Alpert, J., and E. Charney. 1973. *The education of physicians for primary care.* Washington, DC: US DHEW.

Alster, K.B. 1989. *The holistic health movement.* Tuscaloosa, Alabama: The University of Alabama Press.

American Medical Association Council on Ethical and Judicial Affairs. 1995. "Ethical issues in managed care." *Journal of the American Medical Association* 273: 330–5.

American Nurses' Association. 1997. "Implementing nursing's report card: A study of RN staffing, length of stay and patient outcomes." Washington, DC.

Anderson, R.A., and R.R. McDaniel. 1999. "RN participation in organizational decision making and improvements in resident outcomes." *Health Care Management Review* 24: 7–16.

Arborelius, E., and S. Bremberg. 1992. "What can doctors do to achieve a successful consultation? Videotaped interviews analyzed by the 'consultation map' method." *Family Practice* 9: 61–6.

– and K.D. Thakker. 1995. "Why is it so difficult for general practitioners to discuss alcohol with patients?" *Family Practice* 12: 419–22.

Arnould, E., and L. Price. 1993. "River magic: Extraordinary experience and the extended service encounter." *Journal of Consumer Research* 20: 24–45.

Ashforth, B.E., and R.H. Humphrey. 1993. "Emotional labor in service roles: The influence of identity." *Academy of Management Review* 18: 88–115.

Backman, L., and B. Molander. 1986. "Effects of adult age and level of skill on the ability to cope with high-stress condition in a precision sport." *Psychology and Aging* 1: 334–6.

Bain, D. 1979. "The relationship between time and clinical management in family practice." *Journal of Family Practice* 8: 551–9.

Barr, D.A. 1995. "The effects of organizational structure on primary care outcomes under managed care." *Annals of Internal Medicine* 122: 353–9.

Barrera Jr, M., I.N. Sandler, and T.B. Ramsay. 1981. "Preliminary development of a scale of social support: Studies on college students." *American Journal of Community Psychology* 9: 435–47.

Barton, S. 1994. "Chaos, self-organization, and psychology." *American Psychologist* 49: 5–14.

Becker, M.H., R.H. Drachman, and J.P. Kirscht. 1974. "A field experiment to evaluate various outcomes of continuity of physician care." *American Journal of Public Health* 64: 1,062–70.

Beckman, H.B., and R.M. Frankel. 1984. "The effect of physician behavior on the collection of data." *Annals of Internal Medicine* 101: 692–6.

– K.M. Markakis, A.L. Suchman, and R.M. Frankel. 1994. "The doctor-patient relationship and malpractice: Lessons from plaintiff depositions." *Archives of Internal Medicine* 154: 1,365–70.

Behner, K.G., L.F. Fogg, L.C. Fournier, J.T. Frankenbach, and S.B. Robertson. 1990. "Nursing resource management: Analyzing the relationship between costs and quality in staffing decisions." *Health Care Management Review* 15: 63–71.

Bensing, J. 1991. "Doctor-patient communication and the quality of care: An observation study into affective and instrumental behavior in general practice." *Social Science Medicine* 32: 1,301–10.

Ben-Sira, Z. 1976. "The function of the professional's affective behavior in client satisfaction: A revised approach to social interaction theory." *Journal of Health and Social Behavior* 17: 3–11.

– 1980. "Affective and instrumental components in the physician-patient relationship: An additional dimension of interaction theory." *Journal of Health and Social Behavior* 21: 170–80.

Berkowitz, L. 1993. "Towards a general theory of anger and emotional aggression: Implications of the cognitive neoassociationistic perspective for the analysis of anger and other emotions." In R.S. Wyer and T.K. Srull, eds, *Advances in Social Cognition*. Hillsdale, New Jersey: Erlbaum.

Berliner, H., and W.J. Salmon. 1980. "The holistic alternative to scientific medicine: History and analysis." *International Journal of Health Services* 10: 133–47.

Bernard, L.C., and E. Krupat. 1994. "*Health psychology: Biopsychosocial factors in health and illness*." New York: Harcourt Brace.

Blackwell, B. 1996. "From compliance to alliance: A quarter century of research." *Netherlands Journal of Medicine* 48: 140–9.

Blum, R.H. 1957. *The psychology of malpractice suits*. San Francisco: California Medical Association.

– 1960. *The management of the doctor-patient relationship*. New York: McGraw Hill.

Boon, H. 1998a. "The holistic and scientific orientations of Canadian naturopathic practitioners." *Social Science and Medicine* 46: 1,213–25.

– and M. Stewart. 1998b. "Patient-physician communication assessment instruments: 1986 to 1996 in review." *Patient Education and Counseling* 35: 161–76.

Brain, K., P. Norman, J. Gray, and R. Mansel. 1999. "Anxiety and adherence to breast self-examination in women with a family history of breast cancer." *Psychosomatic Medicine* 61: 181–7.

British Medical Association. 1986. *Alternative therapy*. London: The Chameleon Press Limited.

Brown, J.B., and M.E. Adams. 1992. "Patients as reliable reporters of medical care process." *Medical Care* 30: 400–11.

Brown, T., and A. Kirmani. 1999. "The influence of preencounter affect on satisfaction with an anxiety-provoking service encounter." *Journal of Service Research* 1: 333–46.

Buller, M.K., and D.B. Buller. 1987. "Physicians' communication style and patient satisfaction." *Journal of Health and Social Behavior* 28: 375–88.

Burgoon, J.K., M. Pfau, R. Parrott, T. Birk, R. Coker, and M. Burgoon. 1987. "Relational communication, satisfaction, compliance-gaining strategies, and compliance in communication between physicians and patients." *Communication Monographs* 54: 307–24.

Burns, M.O., and M.E.P. Seligman. 1991. "Explanatory style, helplessness, and depression." In C.R. Snyder and R.F. Donelson, eds., *Handbook of Social and Clinical Psychology: The Health Perspective*. New York: Pergamon Press.

Busemeyer, J.R., and J.T. Townsend. 1993. "Decision field theory: A dynamic-cognitive approach to decision making in an uncertain environment." *Psychological Review* 100: 432–59.

Cairney, R. 1997. "Health care as an election issue: Alberta's experience." *Canadian Medical Association Journal* 156: 1,438–40.

Canadian Nurses Association. 1997. "The future supply of registered nurses." Ottawa.

Caplan, G. 1974. *Support systems and community mental health: Lectures on concept development*. New York: Behavioral Publications.

Carstensen, L.L., and S. Turk-Charles. 1994. "The salience of emotion across the adult life span." *Psychology and Aging* 9: 259–64.

Cecil, D.W. 1998. "Relational control patterns in physician-patient clinical encounters: Continuing the conversation." *Health Communications* 10: 125–49.

Charney, E., R. Bynum, D. Eldridge, D. Frank, J.B. MacWhinney, N. McNabb, et al. 1967. "How well do patients take oral penicillin? A collaborative study in private practice." *Pediatrics* 40: 188–95.

Clement, D.G., S.M. Retchin, R.S. Brown, and M.H. Stegall. 1994a. "Access and outcomes of elderly patients enrolled in managed care." *Journal of the American Medical Association* 271: 1,487–92.

– S.M. Retchin, and R.S. Brown. 1994b. "Satisfaction with access and quality of care in Medicare risk contract HMOs." In H.S. Luft, ed., HMOs *and the Elderly*. Ann Arbor, MI: Health Administration Press.

Clinical Quality Improvement Network (CQIN) investigators. 1995. "Low incidence of assessment and modification of risk factors in acute care patients at high risk for cardiovascular events, particularly among females and the elderly." *American Journal of Cardiology* 76: 570–3.

– 1996. "Mortality risk and patterns of practice in 4,606 acute care patients with congestive heart failure: The relative importance of age, sex and medical therapy." *Archives of Internal Medicine* 156: 1,669–73.

Cobb, S. 1976. "Social support as a moderator of life stress." *Psychosomatic Medicine* 38: 300–14.

Cohen, S., and H.M. Hoberman. 1983. "Positive events and social support as buffers of life change stress." *Journal of Applied Social Psychology* 13: 99–125.

Cole, A. 1992. "High anxiety." *Nursing Times* 88: 26–30.

Conger, J.A., and R.N. Kanungo. 1988. "The empowerment process: Integrating theory and practice." *Academy of Management Review* 13: 471–82.

Côté, S., and D.S. Moskowitz. 1998. "On the dynamic covariation between interpersonal behaviour and affect: Prediction from neuroticism, extraversion, and agreeableness." *Journal of Personality and Social Psychology* 75: 1,032–46.

Cox, J.L., on behalf of the ICONS investigators. 1999. "Optimizing disease management at a health care system level: The Improving Cardiovascular Outcomes in Nova Scotians (ICONS) study." *Canadian Journal of Cardiology* 15: 787–96.

Cronbach, L. 1970. *Essentials of psychological testing*. New York: Harper and Row Publishers.

CTV/Angus Reid Group. 1997 (August). "Use of alternative medicines and practices." Winnipeg: Angus Reid Group.

Cutrona, C.E. 1986. "Behavioral manifestations of social support: A micro-analytic investigation." *Journal of Personality and Social Psychology* 51: 201–8.

Davidson, H., P.H. Folcarelli, S. Crawford, L.J. Duprat, and J.C. Clifford. 1997. "The effects of health care reforms on job satisfaction and voluntary turnover among hospital-based nurses." *Medical Care* 35: 634–45.

Davies, A.R., J.E. Ware Jr, R.H. Brook, J.R. Peterson, and J.P. Newhouse. 1986. "Consumer acceptance of prepaid and fee-for-service medical care: Results from a randomized controlled trial." *Health Services Research* 21: 429–52.

– and J.E. Ware Jr. 1988. "Involving consumers in quality of care assessment." *Health Affairs (Millwood)*: 33–48.

Deckard, G., M. Meterko, and D. Field. 1994. "Physician burnout: An examination of personal, professional, and organizational relationships." *Medical Care* 32: 745–54.

Delbanco, T., D.M. Berwick, J[di] Boufford, S. Edgman-Levitan, G. Ollenschläger, D. Plamping, and R.G. Rockefeller. 2001. "Healthcare in a land called PeoplePower: Nothing about me without me." *Health Expectations* 4: 144–50.

Deptula, D., R. Singh, and N. Pomara. 1993. "Aging, emotional states, and memory." *American Journal of Psychiatry* 150: 429–34.

Diefenbach, M.A., E.A. Leventhal, H. Leventhal, and L. Patrick-Miller. 1996. "Negative affect relates to cross-sectional but not longitudinal symptom reporting: Data from elderly adults." *Health Psychology* 15: 282–8.

Dillman, D.A. 1978. *Mail and telephone surveys: The total design method.* New York: John Wiley.

– 1991. "The design and administration of mail surveys." *Annual Review of Sociology* 17: 225–49.

Di Matteo, M.R. 1994. "Enhancing patient adherence to medical recommendations." *Journal of the American Medical Association* 271: 79–83.

– 1995. "Patient adherence to pharmacotherapy: The importance of effective communication." *Formulary* 30: 596–8, 601–2, 605.

– L.M. Prince, and A. Taranta. 1979. "Patients' perceptions of physicians' behavior: Determinants of patient commitment to the therapeutic relationship." *Journal of Community Health* 4: 280–90.

– and R.D. Hays. 1980. "The significance of patients' perceptions of physician conduct: A study of patient satisfaction in a family practice center." *Journal of Community Health* 6: 18–34.

– and D.D. Di Nicola. 1982. *Achieving patient compliance*. New York: Pergamon Press.

– L.S. Linn, B.L. Chang, and D.W. Cope. 1985. "Affect and neutrality in physician behavior: A study of patients' values and satisfaction." *Journal of Behavioral Medicine* 8: 397–410.

– C.D. Sherbourne, R.D. Hays, L. Ordway, R.L. Kravitz, E.A. McGlynn, et al. 1993. "Physicians' characteristics influence patients' adherence to medical treatment: Results from the Medical Outcomes Study." *Health Psychology* 12: 93–102.

– and H.S. Lepper. 1998. "Promoting adherence to courses of treatment: Mutual collaboration in the physician-patient relationship." In L.D. Jackson, B.K. Duffy, et al., eds, *Health Communication Research: A Guide to Developments and Directions*. Westport, CT: Greenwood.

Dracup, K., D.K. Moser, M. Eisenberg, H. Meischke, A.A. Alonzo, and A. Braslow. 1995. "Causes of delay in seeking treatment for heart attack symptoms." *Social Science & Medicine* 40: 379–92.

Dubé, L., M.C. Bélanger, and E. Trudeau. 1996a. "The role of emotions in healthcare satisfaction." *Journal of Healthcare Marketing* 16: 45–51.

– and M.S. Morgan. 1996b. "Trend effects and gender differences in retrospective judgements of consumption emotions." *Journal of Consumer Research* 23: 156–62.

– K. Jedidi, and K. Menon. 1997. "Linking satisfaction to the in-process evolution of consumer emotions and perceived service quality." Denver, Colorado: Association for Consumer Research Conference.

– and M.S. Morgan. 1998a. "Capturing the dynamics of in-process consumption emotions and satisfaction in extended service transactions." *International Journal of Research in Marketing* 15: 309–20.

– and K. Menon. 1998b. "Managing emotions: Accenting the positive might not produce the highest satisfaction payoff." *Marketing Health Services* 18: 34–42.

– M. Johnson, and L. Renaghan. 1999. "Adapting the QFD approach to extended service transactions." *Production and Operations Management* 8: 301–17.

– L. Teng, J. Hawkins, and M. Kaplow. 2002. "Emotions: The neglected side of patient-centered care." In C. Blair Savage and M. Fottler, eds, *Advances in Health Care Management*. Vol. 3. UK: Elsevier Science Ltd.

Duncan, S.M., K. Hyndman, C.A. Estabrooks, K.L. Hesketh, C.K. Humphrey, J.S. Wong, S. Acorn, and P. Giovanetti. 2001. "Nurses' experience of violence in Alberta and British Columbia hospitals." *Canadian Journal of Nursing Research* 32, no. 4: 57–78.

Dworkin, J., G. Albrecht, and J. Cooksey. 1991. "Concerns about AIDS among hospital physicians, nurses and social workers." *Social Science & Medicine* 33: 239–48.

Eisenberg, D.M., R.B. Davis, S.L. Ettner, et al. 1998. "Trends in alternative medicine use in the United States, 1990–1997: Results of a follow-up national survey." *Journal of the American Medical Association* 280: 1,569–75.

Emanuel, E.J., and N.N. Dubler. 1995. "Preserving the physician-patient relationship in the era of managed care." *Journal of the American Medical Association* 273: 323–9.

Engel, G.L., 1977. "The need for a new medical model: A challenge for biomedicine." *Science* 196: 129–36.

Eraker, S.A., J.P. Kirscht, and M.H. Becker. 1984. "Understanding and improving patient compliance." *Annals of Internal Medicine* 100: 258–68.

Estabrooks, C.A., A.E. Tourangeau, C.K. Humphrey, K.L. Hesketh, P. Giovanetti., D. Thomson, J.S. Wong, S. Acorn, H. Clarke, and J. Shamian. 2002. "Measuring the hospital practice environment: A Canadian context." *Research in Nursing and Health* 25: 256–68.

Everson, S. 1997. "Losing your cool can be dangerous to your health." *American Heart Association's 70th Scientific Sessions*. Personal communication.

Falik, M.M., and K. Scott. 1996. *Women's health: A commonwealth fund survey*. Baltimore: John Hopkins University Press.

Felton, J.S. 1998. "Burnout as a clinical entity: Its importance in health care workers." *Occupational Medicine* 48: 237–50.

Ferketich, A.K., J.A. Schwartzbaum, D.J. Frid, and M.L. Moeschberger. 2000. "Depression as an antecedent to heart disease among women and men in the NHANES I Study." *Archives of Internal Medicine* 160: 1,261–8.

Ferris, T.G. 1998. "Today's primary care doctors offer more time and counselling to children but also prescribe more medications." AHCPR 217: 8–9.

Folkman, S., and R.S. Lazarus. 1985. "If it changes it must be a process: Study of emotion and coping during 3 stages of a college examination." *Journal of Personality and Social Psychology* 48: 150–70.

– R.S. Lazarus, and C. Dunkel-Schetter. 1986. "Dynamics of a stressful encounter: Cognitive appraisal, coping and encounter outcomes." *Journal of Personality and Social Psychology* 50: 992–1,003.

– and R.S. Lazarus. 1988. "Coping as a mediator of emotion." *Journal of Personality and Social Psychology* 54: 466–75.

Fournier, M.A., and D.S. Moskowitz. 2000. "The mitigation of interpersonal behaviour." *Journal of Personality and Social Psychology* 79: 827–36.

Francis, V., B.M. Korsch, and M.J. Morris. 1969. "Gaps in doctor-patient communication: Patients' response to medical advice." *New England Journal of Medicine* 280: 535–40.

Francis, A.M., L. Polissar, and A.B. Lorenz. 1984. "Care of patients with colorectal cancer: A comparison of a health maintenance organization and fee-for-service practices." *Medical Care* 22: 418–29.

Frankel, R.M. 1995. "Emotion and the physician-patient relationship." *Motivation and Emotion* 19: 163–73.

Frasure-Smith, N., F. Lespérance, and M. Talajic. 1994. "Depression following myocardial infarction: Impact on 6-month survival." *Journal of the American Medical Association* 270: 1,819–25.

– F. Lespérance, and M. Talajic. 1995. "The impact of negative emotions on prognosis following myocardial infarction: Is it more than depression?" *Health Psychology* 14: 388–98.

Freedman, M.B., T.F. Leary, A.G. Ossorio, and H.S. Coffey. 1951. "The interpersonal dimension of personality." *Journal of Personality* 20: 143–61.

Garrity, T.F. 1981. "Medical compliance and the clinician-patient relationship: A review." *Social Science and Medicine* 15E: 215–22.

Gerbert, B., and W.A. Hargreaves. 1986. "Measuring physician behavior." *Medical Care* 24: 838–47.

Gilmour, B. 1994a. "Health cuts rated biggest in history." *The Edmonton Journal*, 26 October, B14.

– 1994b. "Nursing job losses will worsen – UNA." *The Edmonton Journal*, 21 November, B2.

Goldstein, M.S., C. Sutherland, D.T. Jaffe, and J. Wilson. 1988. "Holistic physicians and family practitioners: Similarities, differences and implications for health policy." *Social Science and Medicine* 26: 853–61.

Golin, C.E., M.R. Di Matteo, and L. Gelberg. 1996. "The role of patient participation in the doctor visit: Implications for adherence to diabetes care." *Diabetes Care* 19: 1,153–64.

Gottlieb, B.H. 1978. "The development and application of a classification scheme of informal helping behaviors." *Canadian Journal of Behavioral Science* 10: 105–15.

Gough, H.G. 1967. "Nonintellectual factors in the selection and evaluation of medical students." *Journal of Medical Education* 42: 642–50.

Government of Canada. 1957. *Hospital insurance and diagnostic services act.* Ottawa.

– 1984. *Canada health act.* Ottawa.

– 1996. *Canada health and social transfer act.* Ottawa.

Grant, M., and M. Tiessen. 1995. "Not a business matter." *Canadian Nurse* 91: 55–7.

Gray, R.E., M. Greenberg, M. Fitch, N. Parry, M.S. Douglas, and M. Labrecque. 1997. "Perspectives of cancer survivors interested in unconventional therapies." *Journal of Psychosocial Oncology* 15: 149–71.

Greenberg, P.E., R.C. Kessler, T.L. Nells, S.N. Finkelstien, and E.R. Berndt. 1996. "Depression in the workplace: An economic perspective." In J.P. Feighner and W.F. Boyers, eds, *Selective Serotonin Reuptake Inhibitors.* Chichester: John Wiley & Sons.

Greenfield, S., S.H. Kaplan, and J.E. Ware Jr. 1985. "Expanding patient involvement in care: Effects on patient outcomes." *Annals of Internal Medicine* 102: 520–8.

– S.H. Kaplan, J.E. Ware Jr, E.M. Yano, and H.J. Frank. 1988. "Patients' participation in medical care: Effects on blood sugar control and quality of life in diabetes." *Journal of General Internal Medicine* 3: 448–57.

Gross, J.J., L.L. Carstensen, J. Tsai, C.G. Skorpen, and A.Y.C. Hsu. 1997. "Emotion and aging: Experience, expression and control." *Psychology and Aging* 12: 590–9.

Hackman, J.R., and G.R. Oldham. 1980. *Work redesign*. Reading, MA: Addison-Wesley.

Hall, J.A., T.S. Stein, D.L. Roter, and N. Rieser. 1999. "Inaccuracies in physicians' perceptions of their patients." *Medical Care* 37: 1,164–8.

– and D.L. Roter. 2002. "Do patients talk differently to male and female physicians? A meta-analytic review." *Patient Education and Counseling* 48: 217–24.

Hayes-Bautista, D.E. 1976. "Modifying the treatment: Patient compliant, patient control, and medical care." *Social Science and Medicine* 10: 233–8.

Hays, R.D., and T. Hayashi. 1990. "Beyond internal consistency: Rationale and user's guide for multitrait analysis program (MAP) on the microcomputer." *Behavioral Research Methods, Instruments, and Computers* 22: 167–75.

Helmers, K.F., and A. Mente. 1999. "Alexithymia and health behaviours in healthy male volunteers." *Journal of Psychosomatic Research* 47: 635–45.

Henbest, R.J., and G.S. Fehrsen. 1992. "Patient-centeredness: Is it applicable outside the west? Its measurement and effect on outcomes." *Family Practice* 9: 311–17.

Hesketh, K.L., S.M. Duncan, C.A. Estabrooks, M.A. Reimer, P. Giovanetti, K. Hyndman, and S. Acorn. Forthcoming. "Workplace violence in Alberta and British Columbia hospitals." *Health Policy*.

Hewer, W. 1983. "The relationship between the alternative practitioner and his patient." *Psychotherapy and Psychsomatics* 40: 172–80.

Hickson, G.B., E.W. Clayton, P.B. Githens, and F.A. Sloan. 1992. "Factors that prompted families to file medical malpractice claims following perinatal injuries." *Journal of the American Medical Association* 267: 1,359–63.

– E.W. Clayton, S.S. Entman, C.S. Miller, P.B. Githens, K. Whetten-Goldstein, et al. 1994. "Obstetricians' prior malpractice experience and patients' satisfaction with care." *Journal of the American Medical Association* 272: 1,583–7.

Hirsch, B.J. 1980. "Natural support systems and coping with major life changes." *American Journal of Community Psychology* 8: 159–72.

Hobfoll, S.E. 1988. *The ecology of stress*. Washington, DC: Hemisphere.

Hochschild, A.R. 1979. "Emotion work, feeling rules, and social structure." *American Journal of Sociology* 85: 551–75.

– 1983. *The managed heart*. Berkeley: University of California Press.

– 2003a. *Commercialization of intimate life: Notes from home and work.* Berkeley and Los Angeles: University of California Press.

– and Barbara Ehrenreich, eds. 2003b. *Global woman: Nannies, maids and sex workers in the new economy.* New York: Metropolitan Press.

Hoffman, C., D. Rice, and H.Y. Sung. 1996. "Persons with chronic conditions: Their prevalence and costs." *Journal of the American Medical Association* 276: 1,473–9.

Holland, T.P., A. Konick, W. Buffum, et al. 1981. "Institutional structure and resident outcomes." *Journal of Health and Social Behavior* 22: 433–44.

Hornberger, J., D. Thorn, and T. MaCurdy. 1997. "Effects of a self-administered previsit questionnaire to enhance awareness of patients' concerns in primary care." *Journal of General Internal Medicine* 12: 597–606.

Horowitz, L.M., L.E. Alden, J.S. Wiggins, and A.L. Pincus. 2000. *Inventory of interpersonal problems manual.* San Antonio, TX: Psychological Corporation.

House, J.S. 1981. *Work, stress, and social support.* Reading, MA: Addison-Wesley.

Howard, K., and G. Forehand. 1962. "A method for correcting item-total correlations for the effect of relevant item inclusion." *Educational Psychological Measures* 22: 731.

Howie, J.G.R., A.M.D. Porter, D.J. Heaney, and J.L. Hopton. 1991. "Long to short consultation ratio: A proxy measure of quality of care for general practice." *British Journal of General Practice* 41: 48–54.

Hull, F.M., and F.S. Hull. 1984. "Time and the general practitioner: The patient's view." *Journal of the Royal College of General Practitioners* 34: 71–5.

Institute of Medicine. 1978. "Report of a study: A manpower policy for primary health care." Washington, DC: National Academy of Sciences.

– 1994. "Defining primary care: An interim report." Washington, DC: National Academy Press.

– 1996. "Primary care: America's health in a new era." Washington, DC: National Academy Press.

Irvine Doran, D.M., and M.G. Evans. 1995. "Job satisfaction and turnover among nurses: Integrating research findings across studies." *Nursing Research* 44: 246–53.

– S. Sidani, and L. McGillis Hall. 1998. "Linking outcomes to nurses' roles in health care." *Nursing Economic $* 16, no. 2: 58–64, 87.

– L. O'Brien-Pallas, S. Sidani, L. McGillis Hall, P. Petryshen, J. Hawkins, and J. Watt-Watson. 2001. "The relationship between patient and system outcomes and the quality of nursing care in acute care hospitals." Final report submitted to the National Health Research and Development Program, Health Canada, Project # 6606–6564–001.

Izard, C.E. 1977. *Human emotions.* New York: Plenum Press.

Jacobson, L.D., C. Wilkinson, and P.A. Owen. 1994. "Is the potential of teenage consultations being missed? A study of consultation times in primary care." *Family Practice* 11: 296–9.

Johns, G. 1996. *Organizational behavior: Understanding life at work.* 3rd edition. New York: Harper Collins.

Johnson, C.G., J.C. Levenkron, A.L. Suchman, and R. Manchester. 1988. "Does physician uncertainty affect patient satisfaction?" *Journal of General Internal Medicine* 3: 144–9.

Kahn, R.L., and T.C. Antonucci. 1981. "Convoys of social support: A life course approach." In S.B. Kiesler, J.N. Morgan, and V.K. Oppenheimer, eds, *Aging: Social Change.* New York: Academic Press.

Kasteler, J., R.L. Kane, D.M. Olsen, and C. Thetford. 1976. "Issues underlying prevalence of 'doctor shopping' behavior." *Journal of Health and Social Behavior* 17: 328–39.

Kaufman, M.R. 1970. "Practicing good manners and compassion." *Medical Insight* 2: 56–61.

Kelso, J.A.S. 2000. "Principles of dynamic pattern formation and change for a science of human behavior." In L. Bergman, R.B. Cairns, L.-G. Nilsson, and L. Nystedt, eds, *Developmental Science and the Holistic Approach.* New Jersey: Erlbaum Associates.

Kessler, R.C., K.A. McGonagle, S. Zhao, C.B. Nelson, M. Hughes, S. Eshleman, H.U. Wittchen, and K.S. Kendler. "Lifetime and 12-month prevalence of DSM-III-R psychiatric disorders in the United States: Results from the National Comorbidity Survey." *Archives of General Psychiatry* 51: 8–19.

Kiesler, D.J. 1996. *Contemporary interpersonal theory and research: Personality, psychopathology, and psychotherapy.* New York: Wiley.

Kjellgren, K[di], J. Ahlner, and R. Saljo. 1995. "Taking antihypertensive medication: Controlling or cooperating with patients?" *International Journal of Cardiology* 47: 257–68.

Klass, P. 1987. *Not an entirely benign procedure: Four years as a medical student.* New York: Signet.

Knaus, W.A., E.A. Draper, D.P. Wagner, and J.E. Zimmerman. 1986. "An evaluation of outcome from intensive care in major medical centers." *Annals of Internal Medicine,* 104: 410–18.

Kocak, H. 1989. *Differential and difference equations through computer experiments.* 2nd edition. New York: Springer-Verlag.

Krantz, D.S., A. Baum, M.V. Wideman. 1980. "Assessment for preferences for self-treatment and information in health care." *Journal of Personality and Social Psychology* 39: 977–90.

Lazarus, R.S. 1990. "Author's response." *Psychological Inquiry* 1: 41–51.

– 2001. "Relational meaning and discrete emotions." In K.R. Scherer, A. Schorr, and T. Johnstone, eds, *Appraisal Processes in Emotion.* New York: Oxford University Press.

– J. Deese, and S.F. Osler. 1952. "The effects of psychological stress upon performance." *Psychological Bulletin* 49: 293–315.

Leary, T.F. 1957. *Interpersonal diagnosis of personality.* New York: Ronald Press.

Lees, M.C., and R.W.J. Neufeld. 1999. "Decision-theoretic aspects of stress arousal and coping propensity." *Journal of Personality and Social Psychology* 77: 185–208.

Lefcourt, H.M., and K. Davidson-Katz. 1991. "Locus of control and health." In C.R. Snyder and R.F. Donelson, eds, *Handbook of Social and Clinical Psychology: The Health Perspective.* New York: Pergamon Press.

Leiter, M.P., P. Harvie, and C. Frizzell. 1998. "The correspondence of patient satisfaction and nurse burnout." *Social Science & Medicine* 47: 1,611–17.

Leopold, N., J. Cooper, and C. Clancy. 1996. "Sustained partnership in primary care." *The Journal of Family Practice* 42: 129–37.

Lespérance, F., and N. Frasure-Smith. 2000. "Depression in patients with cardiac disease: A practical review." *Journal of Psychosomatic Research* 48: 370–91.

Lester, G.W., and S.G. Smith. 1993. "Listening and talking to patients: A remedy for malpractice suits?" *Western Journal of Medicine* 158: 268–72.

Levinson, W., D.L. Roter, J.P. Mullooly, V.T. Dull, and R.M. Frankel. 1997. "Physician-patient communication: The relationship with malpractice claims among primary care physicians and surgeons." *Journal of the American Medical Association* 277: 553–9.

Levenstein, J.H. 1984. "The patient-centred general practice consultation." *South Africa Family Practice* 5: 276–82.

– E.C. McCracken, I.R. McWhinney, M.A. Stewart, and J.B. Brown. 1986. "The patient-centred clinical method: A model for doctor-patient interaction in family medicine." *Family Practice* 3: 24–30.

Lewis, C.E. 1988. "Disease prevention and health promotion practices of primary care physicians in the United States." *American Journal of Preventive Medicine* 4: 9–16.

Ley, P. 1982. "Satisfaction, compliance and communication." *British Journal of Clinical Psychology* 21: 241–54.

– 1985. "Doctor-patient communication: Some quantitative estimates of the role of cognitive factors in non-compliance." *Journal of Hypertension* 3: 51–5.

Linn, L.S., R.H. Brook, V.A. Clark, A.R. Davies, A. Fink, and J. Kosecoff. 1985. "Physician and patient satisfaction as factors related to the organization of internal medicine group practices." *Medical Care* 23: 1,171–8.

Likert, R. 1932. "A technique for the measurement of attitudes." *Archives of Psychology* 140: 1–55.

Lisac, M. 1994. "Bureaucracy is the biggest winner in the Klein revolution." *The Edmonton Journal,* 3 December, A8.

Loyie, F. 1994. "Nursing couple emigrated to U.S. where wife already has secure job." *The Edmonton Journal*, 18 December, B3.

Luft, H.S. 1980. "Assessing the evidence on HMO performance." *Milbank Memorial Fund Quarterly/Health and Society* 58: 501–36.

Lyons, T.F. 1971. "Role clarity, need for clarity, satisfaction, tension, and withdrawal." *Organizational Behavior and Human Performance* 6: 99–110.

Mandelker, J. 1993. "Monitoring drug compliance can reduce total medical plan costs." *Business and Health, Montvale* 11: 26–33.

Marck, P. 1996. "Nurses wary about talk of fewer layoffs: They predict further job losses." *The Edmonton Journal*, 26 January, B3.

Marco, C.A., and J. Suls. 1993. "Daily stress and the trajectory of mood: Spillover, response assimilation, contrast, and chronic negative affectivity." *Journal of Personality and Social Psychology* 64: 1,053–63.

Marvel, K. 1993. "Involvement with the psychosocial concerns of patients." *Archives of Family Medicine* 2: 629–33.

– W.J. Doherty, and E. Weiner. 1998. "Medical interviewing by exemplary family physicians." *Journal of Family Practice* 47: 343–8.

Maslach, C., S.E. Jackson, and M.P. Leiter. 1996. *The Maslach burnout inventory*. 3rd edition. Palo Alto, CA: Consulting Psychologists Press.

Maurier, W.L., and H.C. Northcott. 2000. "Job uncertainty and health status of nurses during restructuring of health care in Alberta. *Western Journal of Nursing Research* 22, no. 5: 623–41.

McCracken, E.C., M.A. Stewart, J.B. Brown, and I.R. McWhinney. 1983. "Patient-centred care: The family practice model." *Canadian Family Physician* 29: 2,313–16.

McGillis Hall, L. 1997. "Staff mix models: Complementary or substitution roles for nurses." *Nursing Administration Quarterly* 21, no. 2: 31–9.

– D.M. Irvine Doran, H. Laschinger, C. Mallette, and L. O 'Brien-Pallas. 2001a. "A component of Hospital Report 2001." Ontario Ministry of Health and Long-Term Care (MOHLTC).

– D.M. Irvine Doran, R. Baker, G. Pink, S. Sidani, L. O'Brien-Pallas, and G. Donner. 2001b. "A study of the impact of nursing staff mix models and organizational change strategies on patient, system, and caregiver outcomes." Final report submitted to the Canadian Health Services Research Foundation and the Ontario Council of Teaching Hospitals.

McKinlay, J.B. 1975. "Who is really ignorant – physician or patient?" *Journal of Health and Social Behavior* 16: 3–11.

Mechanic, D. 1975. "The organization of medical practice and practice orientations among physicians in prepaid and nonprepaid primary care settings." *Medical Care* 13: 189–204.

– 1996. "Changing medical organization and the erosion of trust." *The Milbank Quarterly* 74: 171–89.

– N. Weiss, and P.D. Cleary. 1983. "The growth of HMOs: Issues of enrollment and disenrollment." *Medical Care* 21: 338–47.

Mendlowicz, M.V., and M.B. Stein. 2000. "Quality of life in individuals with anxiety disorders." *American Journal of Psychiatry* 157: 669–82.

Menon, K. 1999a. "Consumer anger and anxiety in airline services." PhD thesis, McGill University, Montreal.

– and L. Dubé. 1999b. "Scripting consumer emotions in extended service: A prerequisite for successful adaptation of provider performance." In E. Arnould and L.M. Scott, eds, "Advances in Consumer Research Conference: Provo." *UT Association for Consumer Research* 26: 18–24.

– and L. Dubé. 2000. "Engineering effective interpersonal responses to customer emotions for higher satisfaction." *Journal of Retailing* 76: 285–307.

– and L. Dubé. 2001. "More than just a feeling: Components of consumer anger and anxiety and their impact on performance evaluation in airline services." Manuscript under review.

Miller, R.H., and H.S. Luft. 1994. "Managed care plan performance since 1980: A literature analysis." *Journal of the American Medical Association* 271: 1,512–19.

Millis, J.S. 1966. *The Millis commission report.* Chicago: American Medical Association.

Mitchell, P.H., S. Armstrong, T.F. Simpson, and M. Lentz. 1989. "American Association of Critical Care Nurses demonstration project: Profile of excellence in critical care nursing." *Heart & Lung* 18: 219–37.

Montague, T. 1999. "Creating a sound clinical basis for health policy: Closing the care gap." In M.A. Somerville, ed., *Do We Care? Renewing Canada's Commitment to Health.* Proceedings of the First Directions for Canadian Health Care Conference. Montreal & Kingston: McGill-Queen's University Press.

– L. Taylor, M. Barnes, M. Ackman, R. Tsuyuki, R. Wensel, R. Williams, D. Catellier, and K. Teo, on behalf of the Clinical Quality Improvement Network (CQIN) investigators. 1995. "Can practice patterns be successfully altered? Examples from cardiovascular medicine." *Canadian Journal of Cardiology* 11: 487–92.

– J. Sidel, B. Erhardt, G. Nakhlé, L. Caron, D. Croteau, M. Kader, J. Haket, K. Skilton, and B. McLeod. 1997. "Patient health management: A promising paradigm in Canadian healthcare." *American Journal of Management Care* 3: 1,175–82.

Montano, D.E., and W.R. Phillips. 1995. "Cancer screening by primary care physicians: A comparison of rates obtained from physician self-report, patient survey, and chart audit." *American Journal of Public Health* 85: 795–800.

Morrison, M.S., R.W.J. Neufeld, and L. Lefebvre. 1988. "The economy of probabilistic stress: Interplay of controlling activity and threat reduction." *British Journal of Mathematical and Statistical Psychology* 41: 155–77.

References 177

Mosher-Ashley, P.M. 1995. "Attendance patterns of elders who accepted counselling following referral to a mental health center." *Clinical Nurse Specialist* 16: 3–19.

Moskowitz, D.S. 1994a. "Cross-situational generality and the interpersonal circumplex." *Journal of Personality and Social Psychology* 66: 921–33.

– E.J. Suh, and J. Desaulniers. 1994b. "Situational influences on gender differences in agency and communion." *Journal of Personality and Social Psychology* 66: 753–61.

– and S. Côté. 1995. "Do interpersonal traits predict affect: A comparison of three models." *Journal of Personality and Social Psychology* 69: 915–24.

Murphy, J., H. Chang, J.E. Montgomery, W.H. Rogers, and D.G. Safran. 2001. "The quality of physician-patient relationships: Patients' experiences 1996–1999." *Journal of Family Practice* 50: 123–9.

Murray, A., and D.G. Safran, W.H. Rogers, T.S. Inui, H. Chang, and J.E. Montgomery. 2000a. "Part-time physicians: Physician workload and patient-based assessments of primary care performance." *Archives of Family Medicine* 9: 327–32.

– and D.G. Safran. 2000b. "The Primary Care Assessment Survey: A tool for measuring, monitoring, and improving primary care." In M.E. Maruish, ed., *Handbook of Psychological Assessment*. Mahwah, NJ: Lawrence Erlbaum Associates, Inc.

Murray, C.J., and A.D. Lopez. 1996. "The global burden of disease in 1990: Final results and their sensitivity to alternative epidemiological perspectives, discount rates, age weights and disability weights." In C.J. Murray and A.D. Lopez, eds, *The Global Burden of Disease: A Comprehensive Assessment of Mortality and Disability from Diseases, Injuries, and Risk Factors in 1990 and Projected to 2020*. Vol. 1. Cambridge, Mass.: Harvard School of Public Health, on behalf of the World Health Organization and the World Bank, distributed by Harvard University Press.

Murray, J.P. 1988. "A follow-up comparison of patient satisfaction among prepaid and fee-for-service patients." *Journal of Family Practice* 26: 576–81.

Musialowski, D.M. 1988. "Perceptions of physicians as a function of medical jargon and subjects' authoritarianism." *Representative Research in Social Psychology* 18: 3–14.

National Institutes of Health (NIH) Panel on Definition and Description. 1995. "Defining and describing complementary and alternative medicine." *Alternative Therapies in Health & Medicine* 3, no. 2: 49–57.

Needleman, J., P. Buerhaus, S. Mattke, M. Stewart, and K. Zelevinsky. 2002. "Nurse-staffing level and the quality of care in hospitals." *New England Journal of Medicine* 346: 1,715–22.

Neufeld, R.W.J. 1999. "Dynamic differentials of stress and coping." *Psychological Review* 106: 385–97.

– and I.R. Nicholson. 1991. "Differential and other equations essential to a servocybernetic (systems) approach to stress-schizophrenia relations." *Research Bulletin* 698. University of Western Ontario, Canada.

Nicholson, I.R., and R.W.J. Neufeld. 1992. "A dynamic vulnerability perspective on stress and schizophrenia." *American Journal of Orthopsychiatry* 62: 117–30.

Nunnelly, J., and I. Bernstein. 1994. *Psychometric Theory.* 3rd edition. New York: McGraw-Hill.

O'Brien, M.T. 1993. "Multiple sclerosis: Stressors and coping strategies in spousal caregivers." *Journal of Community Health Nursing* 10: 123–35.

Olfson, M., M. Guardino, E. Struening, and F.R. Schneier. 2000. "Barriers to the treatment of social anxiety." *American Journal of Psychiatry* 157: 521–7.

Oliver, R.L., 1997. *Satisfaction: A behavioral perspective on the consumer.* New York: McGraw-Hill.

Ormel, J., M. VonKorff, T.B. Ustun, S. Pini, A. Korten, and T. Oldehinkel. 1994. "Common mental disorders and disability across cultures: Results from the WHO collaborative study on psychological problems in general health care." *Journal of the American Medical Association* 272: 1,741–8.

Palfai, T., and K. Hart. 1997. "Anger coping styles and perceived social support." *Journal of Social Psychology* 137: 405–11.

Parkinson, B. 1995. *Ideas and realities of emotions.* New York: Routledge.

Pereles, L., and M.L. Russell. 1996. "Needs for CME in geriatrics." Part 2: "Physician priorities and perceptions of community representatives." *Canadian Family Physician* 42: 632–40.

Peterson, C., M.E. Seligman, and G.E. Vaillant. 1988. "Pessimistic explanatory style is a risk factor for medical illness: A 35-year longitudinal study." *Journal of Personality & Social Psychology* 55: 23–7.

Pinard, G. 1987. "Masked depression: A semantic or diagnostic dilemma." *Annals of the Royal College of Physicians and Surgeons of Canada* 20: 17–20.

– and L. Tétreault. 1974. "Concerning semantic problems in psychological evaluation." *Modern Problems of Pharmacopsychiatry* 7: 8–22.

Prigogine, I., and I. Stengers. 1984. *Order out of chaos.* Colorado: Shambhala Publications.

Putnam, R. 2000. *Bowling alone: The collapse and revival of American community.* New York: Simon & Schuster.

Ramsay, C., M. Walker, and J. Alexander. 1999. "Alternative medicine in Canada: Use and public attitudes." *Public Policy Sources Number 21.* Vancouver: The Fraser Institute.

Reeve, J., E. Bolt, and Y. Car. 1999. "Autonomy-supportive tactics: How they teach and motivate children." *Journal of Educational Psychology* 91: 537–48.

Ridsdale, L., M. Morgan, and R. Morris. 1992. "Doctors' interviewing technique and its response to different booking times." *Family Practice* 9: 57–60.

Roberts, C.A., and M.S. Aruguete. 2000. "Task and socioemotional behaviors of physicians: A test of reciprocity and social interaction theories in analogue physician-patient encounters." *Social Science and Medicine* 50: 309–15.

Ross, C.E., and R.S. Duff. 1982. "Returning to the doctor: The effect of client characteristics, types of practice, and experiences with care." *Journal of Health and Social Behavior* 35: 161–78.

Roter, D.L. 1989. "Which facets of communication have strong effects on outcome: A meta-analysis." In M. Stewart and D.L. Roter, eds, *Communication with Medical Patients*. Newbury Park: Sage.

– and J.A. Hall. 1987. "Physicians' interviewing styles and medical information obtained from patients." *Journal of General Internal Medicine* 2: 325–9.

– J.A. Hall, and Y. Aoki. 2002. "Physician gender effects in medical communication: A meta-analytic review." *Journal of the American Medical Association* 288: 756–64.

Rothenberg, R.B., and J.P. Koplan. 1990. "Chronic disease in the 1990s." *Annual Review of Public Health* 11: 267–96.

Rubin, H.R., B. Gandek, W.H. Rogers, M. Kosinski, C.A. McHorney, and J.E. Ware Jr. 1993. "Patients' ratings of outpatient visits in different practice settings: Results from the Medical Outcomes Study." *Journal of the American Medical Association* 270: 835–40.

Russell, N.K., and D.L. Roter. 1993. "Health promotion counseling of chronic-disease patients during primary care visits." *American Journal of Public Health* 83: 979–82.

Ryan, R.M., and J.A. Solky. 1996. "What is supportive about social support? On the psychological needs for autonomy and relatedness." In G.R. Pierce, B.R. Sarason, and I.G. Sarason, eds, *Handbook of Social Support and the Family*. New York: Plenum Press.

– and E.L. Deci. 2000. "Self-determination theory and the facilitation of intrinsic motivation, social development, and well-being." *American Psychologist* 55: 68–78.

Ryten, E. 1997. *A statistical picture of the past, present and future of registered nurses in Canada*. Ottawa, ON: Canadian Nurses Association.

Safran, D.G. 1994a. *Defining primary care: A background paper prepared for the Institute of Medicine Committee on the Future of Primary Care*. Boston, MA: Tufts-New England Medical Center.

– 2001a. *Primary Care Performance: Views from the Patient: A Background Paper Prepared for the Robert Wood Foundation Meeting on the Future of Primary Care*. Boston, MA: Tufts-New England Medical Center.

– 2003. "Defining the future of primary care: What can we learn from patients?" *Annals of Internal Medicine* 138: 248–55.

– A.R. Tarlov, and W.H. Rogers. 1994b. "Primary care performances in fee-for-service and prepaid health care systems: Results from the Medical Outcomes Study." *Journal of the American Medical Association* 271: 1,579–86.

- W.H. Rogers, J.E. Montgomery, A. Murray, H. Chang, and A.R. Tarlov. 1998a. "Integrating measures of socioeconomic characteristics of patients and their environments into primary care research." Presented at the 126th Annual Meeting of the American Public Health Association, Washington, DC.
- D.A. Taira, W.H. Rogers, M. Kosinski, J.E. Ware Jr, and A.R. Tarlov. 1998b. "Linking primary care performance to outcomes of care." *Journal of Family Practice* 47: 213–20.
- W.H. Rogers, A.R. Tarlov, et al. 1998c. "Organizational and financial characteristics of health plans: Do they affect primary care performance?" *Journal of General Internal Medicine* 13: 66.
- M. Kosinski, A.R. Tarlov, W.H. Rogers, D.A. Taira, N. Lieberman, et al. 1998d. "The Primary Care Assessment Survey: Tests of data quality and measurement performance." *Medical Care* 36: 728–39.
- J.E. Montgomery, W.H. Rogers, A. Murray, H. Chang, and A.R. Tarlov. 1999. "Who are you and where do you live? Social class and sociodemographics as predictors of primary care quality." Presented to the Association for Health Services Research, Chicago, IL.
- A. Murray, H. Chang, J.E. Montgomery, and W.H. Rogers. 2000a. "Linking doctor-patient relationship quality to outcomes." *Journal of General Internal Medicine* 15, supplement 1: 116.
- W.H. Rogers, A.R. Tarlov, T.S. Inui, D.A. Taira, J.E. Montgomery, et al. 2000b. "Organizational and financial characteristics of health plans: Are they related to primary care performance?" *Archives of Internal Medicine* 160: 69–76.
- J.E. Montgomery, H. Chang, J. Murphy, and W.H. Rogers. 2001b. "Switching doctors: Predictors of voluntary disenrollment from a primary physician's practice." *Journal of Family Practice* 50: 130–6.
Sanson-Fisher, R.W., E.M. Campbell, S. Redman, and D.J. Hennrikus. 1989. "Patient-provider interactions and patient outcomes." *Diabetes Educator* 15: 134–8.
Sarason, B.R., I.G. Sarason, and G.R. Pierce. 1990. "Traditional views of social support and their impact on assessment." In B.R Sarason, I.G. Sarason, and G.R. Pierce, eds, *Social Support: An Interactional View.* New York: Wiley.
Saul, J.R. 1998. "Health care at the end of the twentieth century: Confusing symptoms for systems." In M.A. Somerville, ed., *Do We Care? Renewing Canada's Commitment to Health.* Proceedings of the First Directions for Canadian Health Care Conference. Montreal & Kingston: McGill-Queen's University Press.
Sbarbaro, J.A. 1990. "The patient-physician relationship: Compliance revisited." *Annals of Allergy* 64: 325–31.
Scherer, K.R. 1984. "On the nature and function of emotion: A component process approach." In K.R. Scherer and P. Ekman, eds, *Approaches to Emotion.* Hillsdale, New Jersey: Lawrence Erlbaum Associates.

Schumaker, S.A., and A. Brownell. 1984. "Toward a theory of social support: Closing conceptual gaps." *Journal of Social Issues* 40: 11–36.

Schwarzer, R., and A. Leppin. 1989. "Social support and health: A meta-analysis." *Psychology and Health* 3: 1–15.

Scott, R.A., L.H. Aiken, D. Mechanic, and J. Moravcsik. 1995. "Organizational aspects of caring." *Milbank Quarterly* 73: 77–95.

Scott, W. 1968. "Attitude measurement." In G. Lindzey and E. Aronson, eds, *Handbook of Social Psychology*. Vol. 2. Reading, MA: Addison-Wesley.

Sellerberg, A. 1991. "'Hawks' in Swedish medical care: A study of alternative therapists." *Research in the Sociology of Health Care* 9: 191–205.

Sharma, U. 1994. "The equation of responsibility: Complementary practitioners and their patients." In S. Budd and U. Sharma, eds, *The Healing Bond: The Patient-Practitioner Relationship and Therapeutic Responsibility*. New York: Routledge.

Shaver, P., J. Schwartz, D. Kirson, and C. O'Connor. 1997. "Emotion knowledge: Further exploration of a prototype approach." *Journal of Personality and Social Psychology* 52, 1,061–86.

Sherbourne, C.D., R.D. Hays, L. Ordway, M.R. DiMatteo, and R.L. Kravitz. 1992. "Antecedents of adherence to medical recommendations: Results from the Medical Outcomes Study." *Journal of Behavioral Medicine* 15, 447–68.

Sherwood, G., J. Adams-McNeill, P.L. Starck, B. Nieto, and C.J. Thompson. 2000. "Qualitative assessment of hospitalized patients' satisfaction with pain management." *Research in Nursing and Health* 23: 486–95.

Shortell, S.M., J.E. Zimmerman, D.M. Rousseau, R.R. Gillies, D.P. Wagner, E.A. Draper, W.A. Knaus, and J. Duffy. 1994. "The performance of intensive care units: Does good management make a difference?" *Medical Care* 32, 508–25.

Shorter, E. l985. *Bedside manners*. New York: Simon and Schuster.

Sidani, S., and D.M. Irvine Doran. 1999a. "Evaluation of the care delivery model and staff mix redesign initiative: The Collaborative Care Study." Report submitted to the Toronto Hospital.

– and D.M. Irvine Doran. 1999b. "A conceptual framework for evaluating the nurse practitioner role in acute care settings." *Journal of Advanced Nursing* 30: 58–66.

Sidel, J., K. Ryan, and J. Nemis-White. 1998. "Shaping the health care environment through evidence-based medicine: A case study of the ICONS project." *Hospital Quarterly* 2: 29–33.

Siegman, A.W., S.T. Townsend, A.C. Civelek, and R.S. Blumenthal. 2000. "Antagonistic behaviour, dominance, hostility, and coronary heart disease." *Psychosomatic Medicine* 62: 248–57.

Silber, J.H., and P.R. Rosenbaum. 1997. "A spurious correlation between hospital mortality and complication rates: The importance of severity adjustment." *Medical Care* 35: 0S77–92.

Simpson, J., W. Rholes, and J. Nelligan. 1992. "Support seeking and support giving within couples in an anxiety-provoking situation: The role of attachment styles." *Journal of Personality and Social Psychology* 62: 434–46.

Smith, C., and P. Ellsworth. 1985. "Patterns of cognitive appraisal in emotions." *Journal of Personality and Social Psychology* 48: 813–38.

Smith, C.K., E. Polis, and R.R. Hadac. 1981. "Characteristics of the initial medical interview associated with patient satisfaction and understanding." *Journal of Family Practice* 12: 283–8.

Smith, W.G., and D. Buesching. 1986. "Measures of primary medical care and patient characteristics." *Journal of Ambulatory Care Management* 9: 49–57.

Sox, H.C., I. Margulies, and C.H. Sox. 1981. "Psychologically mediated effects of diagnostic tests." *Annals of Internal Medicine* 95: 680–5.

Spiegel, J.S., L.V. Rubenstein, B. Scott, and R.H. Brook. 1983. "Who is the primary physician?" *New England Journal of Medicine* 308: 1,208–12.

Spiegel, M.R. 1967. *Applied differential equations.* New Jersey: Prentice-Hall.

Sprott, J.C., and G. Rowlands. 1995. *Chaos data analyzer: The professional version.* New York: American Institute of Physics.

Squier, R.W. 1990. "A model of empathic understanding and adherence to treatment regimens in practitioner-patient relationships." *Social Science and Medicine* 30: 325–39.

Staddon, J.E. 1984. "Social learning theory and the dynamics of interaction." *Psychological Review* 91: 502–7.

Starfield, B. 1992. *Primary care: Concept, evaluation and policy.* New York: Oxford University Press.

Steiger, J. 1980. "Tests for comparing elements of a correlation matrix." *Psychological Bulletin* 87: 245–51.

Stewart, M. 1995. "Effective physician-patient communication and health outcomes: A review." *Canadian Medical Association Journal* 152: 1,423–33.

– J.B. Brown, H. Boon, J. Galajda, L. Meredith, and M. Sangster. 1999. "Evidence on patient-doctor communication." *Cancer Prevention and Control* 3: 25–30.

Stiles, W.B., S.M. Putnam, S.A. James, and M.H. Wolf. 1979. "Dimensions of patient and physician roles in medical screening interviews." *Social Science Medicine* 13A: 335–41.

Stoll, M., G.F. Hamann, R. Mangold, O. Huf, and P. Winterhoff-Spurk. 1999. "Emotionally evoked changes in cerebral hemodynamics measured by transcranial doppler sonography." *Journal of Neurology* 246: 127–33.

Sullivan, M., A. LaCroix, J. Russo, E. Swords, M. Sornson, and W. Katon. 1999. "Depression in coronary heart disease: What is the appropriate diagnostic threshold?" *Psychosomatics* 40: 286–92.

Sutcliffe, P.A., R.A. Deber, and G. Pasut. 1997. "Public health in Canada: A comparative study of six provinces." *Canadian Journal of Public Health* 88: 246–9.

Svarstad, B.L. 1985. "The relationship between patient communication and compliance." In D.D. Breimer and P. Speiser, eds, *Topics in Pharmaceutical Sciences*. Amsterdam: Elsevier.

Taira, D.A., D.G. Safran, T.B. Seto, W.H. Rogers, M. Kosinski, J.E. Ware Jr, et al. 1997a. "Asian-American patient ratings of physician primary care performance." *Journal of General Internal Medicine* 12: 237–42.

– D.G. Safran, T.B. Seto, W.H. Rogers, and A.R. Tarlov. 1997b. "The relationship between patient income and physician discussion of health risk behaviors." *Journal of the American Medical Association* 278: 1,412–17.

– D.G. Safran, T.B. Seto, W.H. Rogers, T.S. Inui, J.E. Montgomery, et al. 2001. "Do patient assessments of primary care differ by patient ethnicity?" *Health Services Research* 36: 1,059–71.

Tavris, C. 1984. "On the wisdom of counting to ten: Personal and social dangers of anger expression." In P. Shaver, ed., *Review of Personality and Social Psychology*. Beverly Hills, CA: Sage Publications.

Taylor, L., K. Teo, J. Cox, W. Tymchak, G. Tremblay, T. Ashton, D. Alter, and T. Montague. 2000a. "Contemporary physician attitudes and practice patterns in acute myocardial infarction: Results of a large Canadian survey." *Canadian Journal of Cardiology* 16: 156F.

– K. Teo, W. Tymchak, J. Cox, D. Alter, T. Ashton, G. Tremblay, and T. Montague. 2000b. "Treatment differences in elderly patients: Insights from a large Canadian survey on contemporary physician attitudes and practice patterns in acute myocardial infarction." *Canadian Journal of Cardiology* 16: 157F.

Teo, K., J. Burton, C. Buller, S. Plante, D. Catellier, W. Tymchak, V. Dzavik, D. Taylor, S. Yokoyama, and T. Montague, on behalf of the SCAT investigators. 2000. "Long-term effects of cholesterol lowering and angiotensin-converting enzyme inhibition on coronary atherosclerosis: The Simvastatin/Enalapril Coronary Atherosclerosis Trial (SCAT). *Circulation* 102: 1,748–54.

Thoits, P. 1986. "Social support as coping assistance." *Journal of Consulting Clinical Psychology* 54: 416–23.

Thom, D.H., and B. Campbell. 1997. "Patient-physician trust: An exploratory study." *Journal of Family Practice* 44: 169–76.

Tolsdorf, C.C. 1976. "Social networks, support, and coping: An exploratory study." *Family Process* 15: 407–17.

Tosteson, D.C., S.J. Adelstein, and S.T. Carver, eds. 1994. *New pathways to medical education: Learning to learn*. Cambridge, MA: Harvard University Press.

Toynbee, P. 1977. *Patients*. New York: Harcourt Brace.

Trobst, K.K. 1999. "Social support as an interpersonal construct." *European Journal of Psychological Assessment* 15, no. 3: 246–55.

– 2000. "An interpersonal conceptualization and quantification of social support transactions." *Personality and Social Psychology Bulletin* 26: 971–86.

Tronto, J. 1993. *Moral boundaries: A political argument for an ethic of care.* London: Routledge.

Tsuyuki, R.T., K. Teo, R.M. Ikuta, K.S. Bay, P.V. Greenwood, and T. Montague. 1994. "Mortality risk and patterns of practice in 2070 patients with acute myocardial infarction 1987–92: The relative importance of age, sex and medical therapy." *Chest* 105: 1,687–92.

Tugwell, P., K.J. Bennett, D.L. Sackett, and R.B. Haynes. 1985. "The measurement iterative loop: A framework for the critical appraisal of need, benefits, and costs of health interventions." *Journal of Chronic Diseases* 38: 339–51.

United States Congress, Office of Technology Assessment. June 1988. "The Quality of Medical Care: Information for Consumers." OTA-H-386. Washington, DC: US Government Printing Office.

van Dam, F.S.A.M. 1986. "Alternative systems of medicine: Critical notes on the Muntendam Commission Report." In British Medical Association, ed., *Alternative Therapy.* London: The Chameleon Press Limited.

Vaux, A. 1988. *Social support: Theory, research, and intervention.* New York: Praeger.

Ventres, W., and P. Gordon. 1990. "Communication strategies in caring for the underserved." *Journal of Health Care for the Poor and Underserved* 1: 305–14.

Verby, J.E., P. Holden, and R.H. Davis. 1979. "Peer review of consultations in primary care: The use of audiovisual recordings." *British Medical Journal* 1: 1,686–8.

Vincent, C., M. Young, and A. Phillips. 1994. "Why do people sue doctors? A study of patients and relatives taking legal action." *Lancet* 343: 1,609–13.

Waitzkin, H. 1985. "Information giving in medical care." *Journal of Health and Social Behavior* 26: 81–101.

Ware Jr, J.E. 1978a. "Effects of differences in quality of care on patient satisfaction." Proceedings of the 17th Annual Conference on Research in Medical Education. Washington, DC.

– M.K. Snyder, and W.R. Wright. 1976. "Part B: Results regarding scales constructed from the patient satisfaction questionnaire and measure of other health perceptions." In *Development and Validation of Scales to Measure Patient Satisfaction with Health Care Services.* NTIS publication PB: 288–330.

– A. Davies-Avery, and A.L. Stewart. 1978b. "The measurement and meaning of patient satisfaction: A review of the literature." *Health and Medical Care Services Review* 1: 1–15.

– and A.R. Davies. 1983. "Behavioral consequences of consumer dissatisfaction with medical care." *Evaluation and Program Planning* 6: 291–7.

– K.K. Snow, M. Kosinski, and B. Gandek. 1993. SF-36 *health survey: Manual and interpretation guide.* Boston, MA: New England Medical Center.

- M. Kosinski, and S.D. Keller. 1996a. "A 12-item short-form health survey: Construction of scales and preliminary tests of reliability." *Medical Care* 34: 220–33.
- M.S. Bayliss, W.H. Rogers, M. Kosinski, and A.R. Tarlov. 1996b. "Differences in 4-year health outcomes for elderly and poor chronically ill patients treated in HMO and fee-for-services systems: Results from the Medical Outcomes Study." *Journal of the American Medical Association* 276: 1,039–47.
- Watson, D., L.A. Clark, and A. Tellegen. 1988. "Development and validation of brief measures of positive and negative affect: The Panas Scale." *Journal of Personality and Social Psychology* 54: 1,063–70.
- Weiner, B. 1985. An attributional theory of achievement motivation and emotion. *Psychological Review* 92: 548–73.
- Weisman, C.S., and C.A. Nathanson. 1985. "Professional satisfaction and client outcomes: A comparative organizational analysis." *Medical Care* 23: 1,179–92.
- Weiss, R.S. 1974. "The provisions of social relationships." In Z. Rubin, ed., *Doing unto Others.* Englewood Cliffs, NJ: Prentice-Hall.
- Wellin, C., and D.J. Jaffe. 2002. "Clock time versus story time: Narrative dimensions of care for the fragile self." Working paper. Center for Working Families, University of California, Berkeley. Available through Work-Family Researchers' electronic network, Boston College.
- Westcott, R. 1977. "The length of consultations in general practice." *Journal of Royal College General Practitioners* 27: 552–5.
- Wiesner, D. 1989. *Alternative medicine: A guide for patients and health professionals in Australia.* Maryborough, Australia: Kangaroo.
- Wiggins, J.S. 1979. "A psychological taxonomy of trait-descriptive terms: The interpersonal domain." *Journal of Personality and Social Psychology* 37: 395–412.
- 1991. "Agency and communion as conceptual coordinates for the understanding and measurement of interpersonal behaviour." In D. Cicchetti and W.M. Grove, eds, *Thinking Clearly about Psychology: Essays in Honor of Paul E. Meehl.* Minneapolis, MN: University of Minnesota Press.
- 1995. *The interpersonal adjectives scales: Professional manual.* Odessa, FL: Psychological Assessment Resources.
- and K.K. Trobst. 1997a. "Prospects for the assessment of normal and abnormal interpersonal behavior." *Journal of Personality Assessment* 68, special issue: 109–25. Reprinted in J.A. Schinka and R.L. Greene, eds, *Emerging Issues and Methods in Personality Assessment.* New Jersey: Erlbaum.
- and K.K. Trobst. 1997b. "When is a circumplex an 'interpersonal circumplex'? The case of supportive actions." In R. Plutchik and H.R. Conte, eds, *Circumplex Models of Personality and Emotions.* Washington, DC: American Psychological Association.

Williams, G.C., V.M. Grow, Z.R. Freedman, R.M. Ryan, and E.L. Deci. 1996. "Motivational predictors of weight loss and weight-loss maintenance." *Journal of Personality and Social Psychology* 70: 115–26.

Williams, J.E., C.C. Paton, I.C. Siegler, M.L. Eigenbrodt, F.J. Nieto, and H.A. Tyroler. 2000. "Anger proneness predicts coronary heart disease risk: Prospective analysis from the Artherosclerosis Risk In Communities (ARIC) Study." *Circulation* 101: 2,034–9.

Williams, M.A., and L.N. Murphy. 1979. "Subjective and objective measures of staffing adequacy." *Journal of Nursing Administration* 9: 21–9.

Williams, S.J., and M. Calnan. 1991. "Key determinants of consumer dissatisfaction with general practice." *Family Practice* 8, no. 3: 237–42.

Wilson, B.M. 1995. "Promoting compliance: The patient-provider partnership." *Advances in Renal Replacement Therapy* 2: 199–206.

Wilson, P[di], 2000. "Deficit reduction as causal story: Strategic politics and welfare state retrenchment." *Social Science Journal* 37: 97–112.

Wolinsky, F.D., and W.D. Marder. 1983. "Waiting to see the doctor: The impact of organizational structure on medical practice." *Medical Care* 21: 531–42.

Woodward, N.J., and B.S. Wallston. 1987. "Age and health care beliefs: Self-efficacy as a mediator of low desire for control." *Psychology and Aging* 2: 3–8.

Zapka, J., R.H. Palmer, W.A. Hargreaves, D. Nerenz, H. Frazier, and C. Warner. 1995. "Relationships of patient satisfaction with experience of system performance and health status." *Journal of Ambulatory Care Management* 18: 73–83.

Zuroff, D.C., D.S. Moskowitz, and R. Koestner. 2000. "Antecedent and consequences of autonomous motivation in therapeutic, educational, and organizational contexts." Unpublished paper. Dept of Psychology, McGill University.

Contributors

HEATHER BOON, BSCPHM, PHD
Department of Health Administration
Heather Boon is a licensed pharmacist, an Ontario Ministry of Health Career scientist, and an assistant professor in the Department of Health Administration, Faculty of Medicine, University of Toronto. In addition, Professor Boon is cross-appointed to the Department of Family and Community Medicine and the Faculty of Pharmacy, University of Toronto. Professor Boon is co-author of the textbook *The Botanical Pharmacy*, chair of the Canadian Society of Hospital Pharmacists' Task Force on complementary/alternative medicine, and a member of the International Editorial Board of the journal *Focus on Alternative and Complementary Therapies*. Her research focuses on the use of complementary/alternative health care services, including the reasons why patients seek complementary/alternative medicine (CAM), how patients make decisions about CAM, the relationship patients develop with CAM practitioners, and the safety and efficacy of CAM therapies and products.

LAURETTE DUBÉ, PHD
Faculty of Management, McGill University
CIHR-SSHRC *Career Scientist*
Dr Laurette Dubé received her PHD in consumer psychology and services marketing management from Cornell University in 1990. She has an MBA in finance from Ecole des Hautes Etudes Commerciales (HEC) and a BSC in health sciences (nutrition) from Laval University, as well as ten years of experience in hospital management. She is the James McGill professor of consumer psychology and services marketing management in the Faculty of Management at McGill University. She is also a CIHR-SSHRC career scientist whose work in

the health domain focuses on the integration of emotions into various facets of health promotion, disease prevention, and health services management, including web, TV, and print communications, clinical encounters, and systems design and management. Her research has been funded by grant agencies in both the health and the social sciences. Her work on consumption emotions, which combines experimental approaches with the dynamic modelling of emotions (e.g., *Journal of Personality and Social Psychology* 1992, *Journal of Consumer Research* 1996, *International Journal of Research in Marketing* 1998, *Psychometrica* 2002, *Personality and Social Psychology Bulletin* 2002, *Cognition and Emotion* 2003), has contributed significantly to the scientific study of the subjective experience of consumption, its engineering, and its outcomes.

CAROLE A. ESTABROOKS, RN, PHD
Faculty of Nursing, University of Alberta
Carole A. Estabrooks is an associate professor in the Faculty of Nursing at the University of Alberta. Her post doctoral studies were at the Institute for Clinical Evaluative Sciences (ICES) in Toronto. She is a Canadian Institutes of Health Research (CIHR) and Alberta Heritage Foundation for Medical Research (AHFMR) scholar.

Professor Estabrooks' program of research is focused on research dissemination and utilization. She currently holds CIHR and AHFMR grants, examining the utilization of research within the context of pain management practices in adult and paediatric populations, as well as the use of research knowledge at multiple decision making levels. She is also a member of the International Hospital Outcomes Study Consortium, investigating the effects of hospital organization and restructuring on patient and nurse outcomes in several countries.

She has held clinical practice, clinical specialist, and management positions in critical care nursing, and has occupied senior administrative positions, overseeing education, quality, and research.

GUYLAINE FERLAND, PHD
Guylaine Ferland received a PhD in nutrition from the Université de Montréal in 1987 and then completed a three-year postdoctoral fellowship in human nutrition at the USDA Human Nutrition Research Center on Aging at Tufts University in Boston. She is an associate professor in the Department of Nutrition at the Université de Montréal and has been the director of clinical research at the Institut universitaire de gériatrie de Montréal since 1997. She is also an adjunct professor in the School of Nutrition at Moncton University.

Professor Ferland's research focuses on two main areas, namely: (1) vitamin K metabolism during aging and how physiological changes affect dietary requirements, and (2) the nutritional health of geriatric clientele and the factors that contribute to its achievement. Her work has appeared in the main nutrition journals.

In recent years, Professor Ferland has served on the Scientific Consultative Council for the Canadian National Institute of Nutrition and was a member of the External Advisory Panel Government Working Group for the review of policies concerning the addition of vitamins and minerals to foods. In 1999 she served as one of the Canadian representatives on the Dietary Recommended Intake (DRI) Micronutrient Panel (Food and Nutrition Board, Institute of Medicine, NAS).

ARLIE RUSSELL HOCHSCHILD, PHD
Department of Sociology, University of California, Berkeley
Arlie Russell Hochschild is a professor of sociology at the University of California, Berkeley, and co-director of the Center for Working Families. She is the author of *The Managed Heart: The Commercialization of Human Feeling*, a book that introduces the concept of "emotional labour" – i.e., the work of "feeling the right feeling for the job." Professor Hochschild's research interests include the sociology of family, the sociology of gender, and social psychology.

DIANE M. IRVINE DORAN, RN, PHD
Faculty of Nursing, University of Toronto
Diane Irvine Doran is the associate dean of Research and International Relations in the Faculty of Nursing, University of Toronto. She is a co-investigator with the Nursing Effectiveness, Utilization, and Outcome Research Unit, Faculty of Nursing, University of Toronto. Diane Irvine Doran is also a recipient of the Ontario Premiers Research Excellence Award. Her research focuses on health care teams, the evaluation of methods for improving quality in nursing practice, and the design and measurement of nursing-sensitive patient outcomes. One group of studies has focused on methods for improving the quality of health care and promoting patient safety. Within this group of studies, Dr Irvine Doran conducted an evaluation of an intervention designed to teach members of multidisciplinary teams methods for making improvements in clinical practice. She is currently investigating the impact of managed competition on the quality of care and outcomes for nurses and patients in the community setting. A second group of studies has focused on the evaluation of alternative health care provider roles, such as those of nurse practitioners and case managers. A third group of studies is focusing on an evaluation of outcome indicators for assessing the quality of nursing care. Within this group, Dr Irvine Doran is leading a project funded by the Ontario Ministry of Health and Long-Term Care that evaluates the feasibility of instituting data collection of nursing-sensitive outcomes in acute care, home care, long-term care, and complex continuing care. Dr Irvine Doran has published papers on nurses' quality of worklife, the measurement of patient outcomes in the home care and acute care settings, nursing roles and outcome assessment, and quality improvement in the hospital sector.

TERRENCE MONTAGUE, MD, PHD
Department of Patient Health, Merck Frosst Canada & Co.
Terrence Montague graduated from Dalhousie University with a doctorate of medicine in 1972. He is one of Canada's pre-eminent experts in evidence-based health management and outcomes research. Currently, he is executive director of the Department of Patient Health and a member of the Executive Operating Committee at Merck Frosst Canada & Co.

Patient Health has as its primary objective to simulate optimal quality health care and patient outcomes at the best systems' cost by moving towards the practice of comprehensive, seamless, and evidence-based medicine. In his current position, Dr Montague leads a group of more than forty people who have a common mission of fostering the twin goals of enhanced partnerships and outcomes measurements within the health care delivery chain. Current partners include health professionals, government, academia, private and public insurers, and patient advocacy groups across the country.

Previously, Dr Montague occupied a number of academic positions at the University of Alberta, the University of British Columbia, and Dalhousie University. He is the author of more than 300 academic papers and has served on the editorial boards of several medical journals.

Dr Montague is a member of the Canadian Cardiovascular Society, the Canadian Association on Gerontology, the American College of Cardiology, the Royal College of Physicians of Canada, and the Royal Canadian Regiment Association.

D.S. MOSKOWITZ, PHD
Department of Psychology, McGill University
D.S. Moskowitz is a professor of psychology and director of the Clinical Psychology Training Program at McGill University. She is a Fellow of the American Psychological Association, a Fellow of the Society for Personality and Social Psychology, and a past recipient of the James McKeen Cattell Sabbatical Award. She is also a past associate editor of *Personality and Social Psychology Bulletin.*

In recent years, Professor Moskowitz's research has opened up the modelling of fluctuations in social behaviour. She has found that while average levels of social behaviour can be calculated for individuals, focusing on the average level masks considerable regular and predictable variation in social behaviour. She has also characterized the joint fluctuations of social behaviour and affect, identifying types of interpersonal behaviour that are consistently associated over time with pleasant affect and other behaviours that are consistently associated with unpleasant affect. To identify these phenomena, she developed a method that reliably and validly assesses the interpersonal behaviour of individuals as manifested over time and in various situations. This method is finding a wide variety of applications, such as in the study of the social behaviours of health care service providers that promote health related behaviours in patients and the study of the effects of medications on social behaviour and affect.

RICHARD W.J. NEUFELD, PHD
Department of Psychology, Social Science Center,
University of Western Ontario
Richard W.J. Neufeld is a professor of psychology and psychiatry at the University of Western Ontario. He graduated with an MS and PHD in psychology from the University of Calgary.

His substantive research interests include stress-effects on cognitive efficiency and coping; the cognitive neuropsychology of schizophrenia, including brain-imaging; and stress-schizophrenia relations, including stress-related lead-indicators of symptom episodes. He has pioneered formal mathematical modelling in each of these areas. His methodological interests include applied quantitative methods. Professor Neufeld was the first psychologist to be awarded the Joey and Toby Tannenbaum Schizophrenia-Research Distinguished Scientist Award. He is a past recipient of the University of Western Ontario – Faculty of Social Science Research Professorship, has served on several grants committees for the Medical and Social Science Research Council, and is a past chairman of the board of the Ontario Mental Health Foundation.

He is the author or co-author of 111 journal articles and of numerous book contributions, and has served as an associate editor of the *Canadian Journal of Behavioral Science*. Professor Neufeld is currently a senior research fellow of the Ontario Mental Health Foundation and is an associate editor of *Psychological Assessment*.

LAWRENCE R. LEVY is a PHD student in the Department of Psychology in the Clinical Psychology program at the University of Western Ontario. He received an MA in clinical psychology from the University of Western Ontario and an Honours BSC in applied mathematics and psychology from York University. His research focuses on the utilization of non-linear dynamical systems theory (chaos theory) and its diagnostic tools for both quantifying and expounding psychological stress, coping, and psychopathology.

WEIGUANG YAO is conducting post-doctoral work at Queen's University's School of Computing. He graduated with an MSC from the China Institute of Atomic Energy and a PHD in applied mathematics from the University of Western Ontario.

GILBERT PINARD, MD
Department of Psychiatry, Faculty of Medicine, McGill University
Gilbert Pinard is a professor of psychiatry at McGill University and senior psychiatrist at the Allan Memorial Institute, Royal Victoria Hospital. He has been the chairman of the

Departments of Psychiatry at McGill University and the Université de Sherbrooke and was the associate dean of Education at the Université de Sherbrooke. He has been honoured for his clinical work with the Exemplary Psychiatrist Award from the National Alliance for the Mentally Ill and the Quebec Alliance for the Mentally Ill.

Professor Pinard's early research concerned patients suffering from depression. He demonstrated changes in syntactical structures related to affect (e.g., sadness, anxiety, and fatigue) as patients responded to antidepressants. This research led to his current interests in the field of cognitive therapy. A major component of his current research is with obsessive-compulsive patients. He is currently involved in a study pairing a serotonin uptake inhibitor to cognitive therapy for the treatment of obsessive compulsive disorder (OCD). This followed the development of assessment tools to evaluate cognitive structures specific to this disorder as well as therapeutic strategies to improve the outcome of treatment of this difficult disorder. He is a participant in an international working group validating cognitive rating scales concerning OCDs.

DEBRA L. ROTER, DRPH
Department of Behavioral Sciences and Health Education, John Hopkins Bloomberg School of Public Health, Baltimore, Maryland
Debra L. Roter is a professor of health policy and management and associate chair of the Department of Behavioral Sciences and Health Education in the Faculty of Social and Behavioral Sciences. She also holds an appointment of professor in the Department of Medicine in the School of Medicine. Professor Roter received her doctorate from the Johns Hopkins School of Hygiene and Public Health in 1977 and has been a faculty member at Johns Hopkins since 1979. She is the recipient of several awards, including the Society for Public Health Education's Beryl Robots Award in recognition of outstanding contribution to health education research, the American Academy on Physician and Patient Award for Outstanding Research Contributing to the Theory, Practice and Teaching of Effective Health Care Communication, and the Johns Hopkins Golden Apple Award for recognition of excellence in teaching. She serves on the editorial board of several journals and various National Institutes of Health (NIH) grant review panels and foundation commissions.

Professor Roter's primary research focus is the study of physician-patient communication. She has developed a method of process analysis applied to audiotapes of medical encounters that has been widely adopted by researchers, both nationally and internationally. Her studies include basic social psychology research into communication dynamics and interpersonal influence, as well as into health education and health services. Her research includes (1) the clinical investigation of patient and physician interventions to improve the quality of communication and enhance its positive effects on patient health outcomes, and (2) educational applications in the training and evaluation of teaching strategies to enhance physicians' communication skills.

DANA GELB SAFRAN, SCD
The Health Institute, New England Medical Center, Boston
Dana Gelb Safran is director of the Health Institute at New England Medical
Center's Division of Clinical Care Research and an assistant professor in the
Department of Medicine, Tufts University School of Medicine.

Professor Safran's empirical research has emphasized the assessment of primary care performance under different models of health care delivery and the
identification of linkages between key attributes of the doctor-patient relationship and outcomes of care. She is the principal investigator for a national study
of Medicare quality funded by the Agency for Health Care Policy and Research
(AHCPR) and the National Institute on Aging, and for another study funded
by the AHCPR and the Robert Wood Johnson Foundation that is designed to
determine the effect of financial and organizational features of health care
systems on primary care performance. Professor Safran's work to refine the
definition of primary care was reflected in a recent report on that subject by
the Institute of Medicine Committee on the Future of Primary Care. She
pioneered a primary care assessment methodology that measures performance
on each of seven defining elements of primary care. Through invited consul-
tancies with the Commonwealth of Massachusetts, the U.S. Senate Committee
on Labor and Human Resources, the U.S. General Accounting Office, and the
Institute of Medicine of the National Academy of Sciences, she has provided
state and federal policy makers information and analysis requested by each to
address immediate health policy concerns. Dr Safran was previously employed
as a policy analyst at the U.S. Congress Office of Technology Assessment and
the United Hospital Fund. She earned her SCM and SCD in health policy from
the Harvard School of Public Health.

KRISTA K. TROBST, PHD
Department of Psychology, York University
Krista K. Trobst is an assistant professor in the Department of Psychology at
York University, where she teaches health psychology and psychological assessment. She obtained her bachelor of arts degree in psychology in 1989 from
the University of Calgary, where she conducted research in social support
processes. She then attended the University of British Columbia, where she
completed a master's degree in social psychology in 1991 and a PhD in clinical
psychology in 1997. During this time, she developed a theoretical and measurement framework for examining social support processes based on the
Interpersonal Circumplex model. She completed her internship training in psychological and neuropsychological assessment at Yale Medical School and a
postdoctoral fellowship with the National Institute of Health.

Professor Trobst does research and theoretical work on structural models
of personality as they relate to health behaviour and health outcomes.

Index

Note: A page number in italics indicates that the information appears in a figure or table.

abuse, psychological and physical: of nurses, 5, 47–51

access: assessing with PCAS, 13, *14*; care gap, 157–8; characteristics, *18*; and health plan type, *31*, 32

acupuncture practitioners, 105

adherence to treatment: correlation to provider satisfaction, 56; impact on care gap, 156; impact of continuity, 16; impact of emotions, 6, 73; impact of patient–provider relationship, 4, 16, 25–6, *26*, 119–21, 135–7; impact of physician communication skills, 7, 16, 107–8

affect. *See* emotions

age: and chronic disease, 4, 84–6; and drug therapy, 155, 157–8; and emotions, 86; and mental health counselling, 75; and time required for interaction, 107

Alberta: Clinical Quality Improvement Network, 154–5, 159; hospital organization and nurse outcomes, 45–54

alexithymia, 74

alternative medicine. *See* complementary medicine

anger: coping with, 90–1; situations provoking, 89; and stroke, 76

anxiety: causing consultation delay, 6, 75; coping with, 90–1; correlation with patient satisfaction, 87–8;

impact on quality of life, 79–80; link with medical conditions, 76–8; situations provoking, 89

art of care, 3–5

attunement to patient needs, 68–9

behaviours: assessing with ICM, 8, 121–2, 130–1; assessing with SAS-C, 8, 124–6, 128–9; of care providers, 134–7; influenced by people present, 134; influenced by role relationships, 134; fluctuating with emotions, 130, 132, *133*, 134; impact of patient–provider relationship, 116, 135–7; prototypical, 131

biomedicine, 3, 115

breast examinations, 75

British Columbia: hospital organization and nurse outcomes, 45–54

burnout: nurses, 47, 51–4, 103; female physicians, 103

Canada Health Act (1984), 46

Canada Health and Social Transfer Act (1996), 46

care gap: causes, 154; closing, 159; defined, 10, 153–4; identifying, 10; in access, 157–8; in diagnosis, 156; in drug therapy, 155; in patient adherence to treatment, 156; measuring, 154; overall, 158

care provider outcomes: impact of art of care, 4; impact of organizational constraints, 4. *See also* nurses; physicians

care providers: coping with personal
emotions, 80; response to patient
emotions, 85, 92–7; as social sup-
ports, 115, 121. *See also* families;
nurses; physicians
chaos theory. *See* dynamic systems
theory
children: primary care assessment,
13
Chinese medicine, 109
chiropractic, 109
chronic diseases: and age, 4, 84–6;
health and economic impacts, 4, 6,
77–8; importance of interpersonal
processes, 3–4
Clinical Quality Improvement Network, 10, 154–5, 159
communication: and adherence to treatment, 7, 16, 107–8; assessing with
PCAS, 13, *14*, *18*; and culture/race,
35, 74; decline of, *37*, 37–8, 99;
gender differences, 100–4; and health
plan type, 30, *31*, 32, *33*; in typical
therapeutic visit, 99–100, *100*; and
patient outcomes, 7, 30, *33*, 105–6,
108; and patient satisfaction, 7, 105–
6, 118–19; study comparing practitioners to family physicians, 110–13;
and time, 106–7, 113
complementary medicine: defined, 108–9;
patient–provider communication, 7,
105, 109–13; study comparing practitioners to family physicians, 110–13;
use of, 109
compliance. *See* adherence to treatment
complications and provider satisfaction,
56–8
comprehensiveness of care: assessing
with PCAS, 13, *14*, *31*; in Canadian
system, 46
continuity of care: assessing with PCAS,
13, *14*; characteristics, *18*; and health
plan type, *31*, 32; improvement
during late 1990s, 37
continuous quality improvement:
and Improving Cardiac Outcomes
in Nova Scotians project, 159–60;
to close care gap, 159
coping: emotion–focused methods, 90;
with emotions, 80–2; problem–focused
methods, 90; with psychological
stress, 146–8

costs: assessing with PCAS, 13, *14*, *18*;
of chronic diseases, 4; of depression,
6, 77–8; of drug therapy care gap,
158; of patient–provided vs. other
data, 14–15. *See also* financial access
counselling: assessing with PCAS, 13,
14, *18*; and health plan type, *31*
CQIN. *See* Clinical Quality Improvement Network
culture: impact on health care interaction, 35, 74

data: accessibility, 14–15; completeness
in PCAS, 21, 23, 42; costs, 14;
demand for, 42; Likert scaling in
PCAS, 17, *19*, 20–1; measurement
performance of PCAS, 21, 22, 23–4;
and outcomes of care, 15–16; reliability and validity, 15
depression: cost of, 6, 77–8; impact on
quality of life, 79; link with medical
conditions, 6, 76–9, 77, 79
diagnosis: care gap, 156–7
diary studies, 131–2
disability: impact of mental illness,
76–7, 77
disease: impact of emotions, 76
disease burden: care gap, 156–7; and
patient–provider relationship, 38,
39, 84
displacement of feelings, 70–1
drug therapy: example of care gap, 10,
155, 157–8; patient non–compliance
with, 156
dynamic systems theory: described,
9, 138–42; and prevention program
for psychoses, 142–5; and psychological stress and coping, 142, 146–9;
value in analyzing interpersonal
aspects of care, 9–10, 140, 142,
149–50
dysthymia, 77–8

elderly: chronic diseases, 4, 84–6; drug
therapy care gap, 155, 157–8; mental
health counselling, 75; negative emotions, 86; time required for interaction, 107
emotional care: defined, 6, 67–9; of
nurses, 72; obstacles to, 69–72
emotional labour: defined, 6, 67; of
nurses, 70–1

emotions: and age, 86; assessing co–
    fluctuations with behaviours, 130–1;
    basic affective dimensions of, 87–8;
    of care providers, 5, 52–4, 80;
    coping with, 80–2, 89–91; defining
    and measuring, 73–4, 86, 96;
    displacement of feelings, 70–1; of
    families, 80; impact on medical
    conditions, 6, 76; impact on patient
    outcomes, 4, 108; impact on patients'
    interaction with health care, 6, 73–5;
    impact on quality of care, 4, 54, 65,
    85–6; impact on quality of life, 79–
    80; inability to talk about, 74; multi-
    component approach to, 88–92;
    and people present, 134; and role
    relationships, 134; using in evidence-
    based practice, 6–7, 92–7. See also
    specific emotions
emotion scripts, 92–3
empathy, 68
England: hospital organization and
    nurse outcomes, 45–54
esteem: in ICM, 121–2, 122; in SAS-C,
    126; in social support literature, 123
ever–contingent recording studies, 131–2

families: as caregivers, 6, 71, 80; coping
    with emotions, 80; as social sup-
    ports, 115, 121
fear, 6, 75
fees for services, 29
female physicians: relationship with
    patients, 7, 102–4; socialization at
    medical school, 101–2
financial access: assessing with PCAS,
    13, 14; defined, 18; no change
    during late 1990s, 37. See also costs

gender: and appreciation for emotional
    care, 69–70; and depression and
    heart disease, 78; and emotions, 87;
    and interpersonal interactions, 7,
    100–4, 101
Germany: hospital organization and
    nurse outcomes, 45–54
government responsibilities for health,
    46–7
guilt: felt by families, 71

health care restructuring: Alberta, 46–7;
    and decline in patient–provider

relationship, 36–8, 39–41, 103;
    and expectations on family, 71, 80;
    and integration of patient emotions
    in care, 84; and provider job satisfac-
    tion, 66
health insurance: comparison of models,
    29–34
health maintenance organizations, 29–32
health plan types and care perfor-
    mance, 29–34, 42–3
heart disease: and anger, 76; and
    anxiety, 78; care gap, 154–5, 155;
    delay in consultation about, 75;
    and depression, 78, 79; diagnostic
    rates, 157; Improving Cardiac Out-
    comes in Nova Scotians project, 155,
    159–60
herbal medicine, 105, 109
HMOS. See health maintenance organiza-
    tions
holistic care. See "whole person" care
Hospital Insurance and Diagnostic
    Services Act (1957), Canada, 46
Hospital Outcomes Study, 45–54
hospitals: importance of staff satisfac-
    tion, 65–6; social support role, 121;
    staff participation and job satisfac-
    tion, 56. See also organizational
    structure

ICM. See Interpersonal Circumplex
    Model
immunosuppressive drugs: patient non-
    compliance, 156
Improving Cardiac Outcomes in Nova
    Scotians project, 155, 159–60
Independent Practice Association. See
    health maintenance organizations
Institute of Medicine, 13, 25
integration of care: assessing with PCAS,
    13, 14, 18; and health plan type, 31;
    no change during late 1990s, 37
international comparisons: nurses and
    patient outcomes, 47–54
interpersonal care: analyzing with
    dynamic systems theory, 9–10, 140,
    142, 149–50; assessing with PCAS,
    13, 14, 18; assessing with SAS-C,
    121–9; decline during late 1990s, 37,
    37–8; and health plan type, 31;
    importance to patient evaluation
    of provider, 117, 136–7; importance

to patient outcomes, 57–8, 65, 136, 136–7; lack of advancements, 3; and role of provider satisfaction in patient outcomes, 57–8, 65
Interpersonal Circumplex Model: described, 121–2, 122, 132; to assess affect and behaviour, 9, 121–2, 131–2
interscale correlations in PCAS, 21, 23–4

jargon, 118–19
job and career satisfaction: nurses, 5, 47–9, 56–8, 62–3, 64–6; physicians, 40, 56, 65–6

knowledge of patients. See "whole person" care

Likert scaling in PCAS, 17, 19, 20–1, 22
longitudinal study using PCAS: methodology, 24–5; results in terms of changes in primary care relationship, 36–8, 37, 39, 40–1, 42–3; results in terms of organizational characteristics, 29–34; results in terms of outcomes of care, 25–7, 26, 28, 29; results in terms of patient characteristics, 35–6, 43; results in terms of physician characteristics, 34–5, 43
love: in ICM, 121–2, 122; in SAS-C, 126; in social support literature, 123

male physicians: relationship with patients, 7, 104
malpractice claims, 106, 119–20
managed indemnity insurance with fees for services, 29–30, 32
mania, 77
Maslach's Burnout Inventory, 51–2
Massachusetts: study on PCAS, 24–44
massage therapy, 109
measurement: to help close care gap, 159; as value system, 152, 153
medical schools: improvements needed in patient–centred training, 104; socialization of female physicians, 101–2
Medicare, 46
meditation, 109
men: interpersonal interactions, 101, 101; work habits, 101

mental health: consultation delay, 74–5; coping with emotions, 81; link with medical conditions, 76–9
mind–body interventions, 109
mood. See emotions

naturopathy, 105, 109
Nova Scotia, Improving Cardiac Outcomes project, 155, 159–60
nurses: Alberta layoffs, 47, 54; attunement to patient needs, 68–9; autonomy and patient outcomes, 61, 62–3; burnout, 47, 51–4, 103; demographics, 49; job and career satisfaction, 5, 47–9, 56–8, 62–3, 64–6; Ontario study on job satisfaction, 58–64; and organizational structure, 5, 45; providing emotional care, 68–9, 72; specialities and job satisfaction, 48–9; workplace violence, 5, 47, 49–51. See also provider outcomes
Nursing Role Effectiveness Model, 58–9, 59
nursing shortages, 47, 54

obsessive compulsive disorder, 75, 82
Ontario: hospital organization and nurse outcomes, 45–54; nurses' job satisfaction and patient outcomes, 58–64; prevention program for psychoses, 142–5
organizational access: assessing with PCAS, 13, 14; decline during late 1990s, 37; defined, 18
organizational structure: health insurance models, 29–34; impact on art of care, 5; impact on nurse outcomes, 4–5, 45, 47–54, 61, 64; impact on patient outcomes, 4
osteoporosis, 157
outcomes of care. See patient outcomes; provider outcomes

panic disorder, 76
patient–centred care: improvements in training needed, 104; physician and complementary practitioner similarity, 110–11; physician gender differences, 100–2
patient compliance. See adherence to treatment
patient education, 107

patient outcomes: impact of emotional processes, 4, 108; impact of organizational constraints, 4; impact of patient-provider relationship, 4, 7, 16, 25–9, 43–4, 115–16, 119–21, 134–7; impact of physician communication skills, 7, 30, 33, 105–6, 108; impact of provider job satisfaction, 5, 56–8, 64–6; predicted with PCAS, 15–16

patient–physician relationship: correlation to art of care, 5; decline in late 1990s, 36–8, 39–41; gender factors, 7, 102–4; influence of technology, 98; and patient characteristics, 35–6, 43; and physician characteristics, 34–5, 43; power relationships, 100. *See also* patient-provider relationship

patient–provider relationship: assessing, 13, 14, 18, 116–17; basis of primary care, 12–13; duration (longitudinal continuity), 13, 14, 18, 31, 38; and health plan type, 39; impact on patient outcomes, 7, 16, 25, 27, 29, 43–4, 115–16, 119–21, 134–7; importance of communication, 13, 14, 18, 99–100, 113–14; improving, 9; in complementary vs. traditional medicine, 7–8; research into, 116–21, 126, 129; and social–support relationship, 8; visit–based continuity, 13, 14, 18, 31, 37–8, 40. *See also* patient-physician relationship

patients: abusing nurses, 50; adherence to treatment, 4, 6–7, 16, 25–6, 26, 73, 107–8; characteristics of and patient outcomes, 35–6, 43; emotional experience of nursing care, 68; emotions. *See main entry* emotions; expectations, 39–40, 107; feeling of lack of options, 41; as information providers, 14–16; loyalty to physicians, 5; participation in decision-making, 107–8, 118, 135–6; time with physician, 38, 39; trust in providers, 4–5, 16, 18, 30, 37, 37–8

patient satisfaction: assessing, 16, 120–1; correlation with emotions, 87–8; correlation to art of care, 4, 25, 27; correlation to provider satisfaction, 56; impact of patient-provider relationship, 116; impact of physician

communication skills, 7, 105–6, 118–19

PCAS. *See* Primary Care Assessment Survey

physical examinations, 13, 14, 18, 31

physical health: consultation delay, 75; coping with emotions, 81

physicians: ability to provide art of care, 5; assessing with PCAS, 13, 14, 18; characteristics desired by patients, 116–19; characteristics of and patient outcomes, 34–5, 43; communication styles and patient outcomes, 7, 30, 33, 105–6, 108; competence, 117–18; gender factors in patient relations, 7, 101–4; and health plan type, 30–2, 34; as information providers, 15; job and career satisfaction, 40; role in primary care, 12–13; role in therapeutic visit, 100; as team members, 32, 33. *See also* provider outcomes

point–of–service model of care, 29–30, 32

portability of health care, 46

preventive counselling, 13, 14, 18, 31

primary care: assessing, 13, 14, 30; components, 13, 14; defined, 12–3, 30. *See also* Primary Care Assessment Survey

Primary Care Assessment Survey: components, 13, 14, 18; development and testing of, 16–24; and longitudinal observational study, 24–9; and measuring and explaining patient-provider relationship changes in the late 1990s, 36–41; and relating health plan type to outcomes, 29–41, 43; and relating patient characteristics to outcomes, 35–6, 43; and relating physician characteristics to outcomes, 34–5, 43; rationale for using patient–provided data, 14–16; value, 42–4

providers. *See* care providers

psychoses: Ontario prevention program, 142–5

public administration of health care, 46

quality of care: assessing with PCAS, 13, 14; impact of emotions, 4, 54, 65, 85–6; impact of nurses' job satisfaction, 64–6; and patients as

information providers, 14–16; relatively recent research concern, 115; technical aspects, 15
quality of life, 79–80
Quebec: community care, 80; prescription drug formulary, 157

race: impact on health care interaction, 35, 74
Reiki, 109
research: degrees of certainty about results, 152, *153*; international study on hospital organization and nurse outcomes, 45–54; into affect and behaviour fluctuations, 131–4; into patient–provider relationship, 116–21, 126, 129; into social support, 121–3; Massachusetts study on PCAS, 24–44; need to understand underlying values, 10; Ontario study on job satisfaction, 58–64; study on patient emotions, provider responses, and care outcomes, 94–6; to enable evidence-based interpersonal care, 151, 153; types in social sciences, 140–2, *141*; using dynamic systems theory, 138–42, 149–50

SAS-C. *See* Support Actions Scale Circumplex
schizophrenia, 142–3
science: importance of integration with art of care, 3–4
Scotland: hospital organization and nurse outcomes, 45–54
seniors. *See* elderly
Simvastatin/Enalapril Coronary Atherosclerosis Trial, 156
social support: for coping with emotions, 81; defined, 121; impact on patient outcomes, 8, 121
sociodemographics: and patient outcomes, 34–6, 43, 75; and time required for interaction, 107
staffing resources: impact on emotional exhaustion, 5

static systems research, 140–1, *141*
status. *See* esteem
stress: and coping, 146–8
stroke: and anger, 76; and depression, 78
Support Actions Scale Circumplex: described, 122–5, *124*, *127*; to assess patient–provider relationship, 125–6, *128*, 128–9; to assess social-support behaviours, 8, 125–6

technology: degrading therapeutic relationship, 98, 115; improving health status, 3, 115
teenagers: time required for interaction, 107
therapeutic touch, 109
time for care: complementary practitioners, 109, 113; nurses, 62–3, 64, 70; physicians, 38, 39, 106–7, 113
trust: assessing with PCAS, 13, 14, *18*; correlation to outcomes, 4–5, 16, 25–9; decline during late 1990s, 37, 37–8; and health plan type, 30, *31*

United States: cost of depression, 77; drug therapy costs vs. overall health system costs, 158; hospital organization and nurse outcomes, 45–54; longitudinal study using PCAS, 24–44; nurses' migration to, 49
universality of health care, 46

violence against nurses, 5, 47–51

"whole person" care: assessing with PCAS, 13, 14, 31; basis of primary care, 12; characteristics, *18*; and complementary practitioners, 112–13; correlation to outcomes, 4–5, 16, 25–9; and health plan type, 30, *31*, 32, *33*; improvement during late 1990s, 37, 37
women: and appreciation for emotional care, 69–70; interpersonal interactions, *101*, 101; work habits, 101

3